Evans Modern Teaching

Learning about Life

Evans Modern Teaching

Learning about Life

A child-centred approach to sex
education

Mary Lane

Evans Brothers Limited London

Published by Evans Brothers Limited
Montague House,
Russell Square, London WC1

Filmset in 11 on 12 pt Imprint by
Photoprint Plates Ltd., Rayleigh, Essex,
and printed in Great Britain by
T. & A. Constable Ltd., Edinburgh

ISBN 0 237 28619 X   PRA 3750

Contents

Introduction

Until recent years the word 'sex' was used to denote gender. Those of us now in middle age probably only used the word ourselves in the context of biology and other natural sciences when we were in school. Today, however, sex has become an umbrella word loosely used by all age groups in conversation on subjects related to sexual drives and response and the different modes of human behaviour between the sexes. It is used descriptively in phrases, 'Sexy clothes, sexy films', and as a statement of fact, 'To have sex'. This common and accepted use of the phrase has led to a change of terminology in schools and we have come round to using the plain phrase 'sex education' rather than, for instance, the subject headings health education, human biology or human physiology, under which labels it was previously hidden.

This use of the word 'sex' to denote an area of the curriculum understandably causes some people concern. The changes in sexual *mores* and open discussion on a previously taboo subject have come rapidly and many responsible adults feel anxiety in the face of increased illegitimacy rates, particularly in young girls, increase in abortion and venereal disease, and in all changes associated with the phrase 'permissive society'. They somehow feel that sex education is part of this trend. This, however, is not true. Its development as part of the secondary school curriculum, and then of the primary school, goes back many years in the work of conscientious teachers whose professional experience gave them an understanding of the needs of young people.

Sex education has been included in the curriculum of different schools at different times for many years according to the personal view of the head and availability of staff to implement learning in accordance with the school's aims.

During and just after the last war pamphlets and reports of the Board of Education and then the Ministry of Education drew attention to the need to consider education in sexual matters at secondary level in both schools and youth clubs.

War-time conditions revealed the ignorance of human sex and venereal disease among national service recruits who had only recently left school.

The 1944 Education Act allowed for development in that

> . . . it shall be the duty of the local education authority for every area, so far as their powers extend, to contribute towards the spiritual, moral, mental and physical development of the community by securing that efficient education shall be available to meet the needs of the population in their area.

Schemes of work in the contexts of biology, health and domestic science, etc., followed in some schools. In some the work was maintained for long periods by heads and staff who acted from the conviction that there was a need which could be met by giving this knowledge in schools. Conversely, in other schools little or no help was given to young people to enable them to learn either the facts of human reproduction, or to understand their own drives and feelings.

Attitudes in society in general did not sufficiently support a definite and organised approach in schools. Indeed even now one still occasionally meets an older teacher who believes that if any words connected with the subject of human reproduction or sex are spoken between teacher and pupil, the teacher is somehow open to suspicion of improper behaviour. Official attitudes in some education circles tended to support this view.

Nevertheless over the years sex education has received thoughtful attention from concerned persons in many different contexts.

It is worth remembering that, as far back as 1930, the Lambeth Conference of Anglican clergy recommended that information on sexual matters should be given in schools before the pupils themselves were emotionally involved, and that such information should be given with simplicity and beauty.

In 1963 Friends Home Service Committee published a thoughtful and thought-provoking essay, 'Towards a Quaker View of Sex', an account of the long deliberations by a group of Friends who were concerned about the predicament of some of their fellow men. This is marked by its open-minded approach and clarity and shows the influence on thinking which the insights from psychology can give us.

In 1964 the Newsom Report of the Central Advisory Council for Education, 'Half Our Future', included these statements based on their assessment of the needs of young people in this area of learning:

1. Boys' and girls' behaviour, confidence and attitude to work can be shaped by successful relations with individual teachers: what ultimately counts is a person.
2. Positive guidance to boys and girls on sexual morals is essential with specific discussion of the problems they will face.
3. Those personal situations which most perplex adolescent boys and girls . . . are situations about which there is no universal contemporary agreement. The challenging feature of their lives is now the sexual instinct which is at its most potent in these years . . . It would be stupid to deny that there are profound differences in society about pre-marital intercourse and about the permanence of marriage, or that these must be reflected in many staff rooms. Tensions there must be if the questions of boys and girls are heard and answered and not suppressed—tensions perhaps within the staff of a school and tension between home and school. We can only say that we believe it to be wrong to conceal from them (as if we could) the differences on this issue which separate men and women of real moral sensitivity.

In 1965 Michael Schofield published an account of his research, 'The Sexual Behaviour of Young People', carried out under the auspices of the Central Council of Health Education with a grant from the Nuffield Foundation. This work revealed most cogently the needs of young people for accurate information and positive guidance. It showed that:

1.   The majority of young people had had no information or guidance on sex from home or school.
2.   That peers were the most likely source of information which was highly inaccurate often due to the over-anxious desire of the purveyors to talk out their own confusions and to pass them on to others.
3.   Knowledge of venereal disease was so limited that they would not be aware of the symptoms and so go for treatment if necessary.
4.   Sexually experienced seventeen- to nineteen-year-olds had a tendency to ethnocentric behaviour. (They tended to a hedonistic view of life with little regard for the views of others. They were little influenced by adult institutions, religion, or moral factors. They were against foreigners, coloured people, the police, homosexuals and marriage.)
5.   Far too little was known of birth control methods and only a very small proportion of young people used them.
6.   A large number of boys (25 per cent) and quite a few girls (13 per cent) were driven towards their first experience for reasons that can best be summed up by the word, curiosity.

Schofield's research was carried out in this country. It revealed the needs of young people leaving our schools. The response to this need has been to attempt to find approaches relevant to the conditions here. Although some of our educationists have studied and considered the work of other countries such as Sweden and parts of the United States, the developments of recent years have been indigenous, to meet conditions in our kinds of schools, our organisations for learning and our way of life.

The developments at secondary level have been largely to widen the concept of sex education to include not only biological and physiological information but provision for discussion through which young people are able to come to an understanding of the complexity and importance of human relationships in all their diversity and be helped to acquire a personal moral code of behaviour. This, on the whole, is most successful when the teacher is known to the young and held in some affection and esteem for innate qualities of personality in addition to those associated with the role of teacher. Such a person is able to guide learning through discussion on a reciprocal basis.

In 1966 a report, 'Sex and Morality', was presented to the British Council of Churches. It included these statements:

1. There is abundant evidence of a deepening concern to provide a more adequate programme of sex education for young people, and to help parents in the discharge of their responsibilities in this field; and this must aim not simply at teaching the biological facts of reproduction (though this is still less efficiently done than is often assumed) but at expressing and conveying a sane and responsible attitude towards love and marriage in the face of the misleading suggestions conveyed by much popular literature, entertainment and advertising.

2. A new, more objective approach is needed in our schools which still have no official place for the communication of that increasing body of knowledge relating to personal relationships, some of it psychological, some sociological, some philosophical and ethical. We would recommend that specific courses on human relations should become part of the curriculum of all schools, introduced at appropriate points up to sixth form level. It is our firm belief that sex instruction should be given within such a context.

3. It is important that more detailed instruction on sexual matters should precede puberty. Physical maturity often comes to the young person unexplained and can cause shock, and even fear. This seems that we must recognise the need for teachers who are prepared to tackle this task in junior as well as secondary schools.

These recommendations were made, among others:

1. Courses on human relations should become part of the curriculum of all schools, and developed at appropriate points up to and including the sixth form.

2. University Institutes of Education should provide courses on human relations which seconded teachers could pursue, perhaps for a recognised qualification.

In 1967 the Central Advisory Council for Education followed their report, 'Half our Future', with the report 'Children and their Primary Schools', under the chairmanship of Lady Plowden. It included these statements:

1. We have no doubt that children's questions about sex ought to be answered plainly and truthfully whenever they are asked.
2. The answers must provide an acceptable and usable vocabulary for the child.
3. Every school must make the arrangements that seem best to it and should have a definite policy, which, in consultation with parents, covers all children.
4. It is not good enough to leave matters vague and open, hoping for the best.

These are sound educational reasons based on an appreciation of the needs of children and the realisation that sex education is part of the wholeness of learning in the school environments described in the Report itself.

But conditions in society today also make it necessary for teachers and other persons concerned with children's welfare to consider the relevance of giving children accurate information to supplement the snippets of information they are able to obtain from television, colour supplements and newspaper headings, and to offer alternative values to those implied by much advertising, some films and film hoardings, paperback covers and magazines.

Many of us have been surprised by the amount of partial knowledge children have revealed by their questions once this part of the curriculum has been opened up by the teacher, and the children have realised that it is something they can learn about if they wish. Twenty years ago, when the writer was first involved in teaching animal and human reproduction, as it then was, to older juniors, it was considered that contraception was quite beyond their interest and understanding. Today, after the process of conception and birth had been understood, the question 'What is the pill a mother can take to stop having a baby?' has been quite common with middle school and junior children. To our knowledge no other form of contraception was asked about. Often the answer to this was followed by, 'But what is the pill that makes a mother have a lot of babies?' We realised from the frequency of the questions, in this order, in different schools, how much children had overheard of adult conversation, television and radio reports and discussions. The fertility pill was current news.

Underlying the changed approach to learning in this field, as in all other areas of knowledge, is our greater understanding of the ways in which learning takes place. Knowledge grows little by little with increased experience, extended vocabulary and a greater understanding of reality. Concepts develop in complexity throughout life and learning starts within hours of birth. We realise that an isolated talk by a school doctor or similar person, a single scheme of work or isolated lesson as a preparation for, or introduction to, a new stage in education and any similar approach which arises from the belief that it is best to get the tricky subject covered quickly and then out of the way to return to a more traditional syllabus, is contrary to children's development and to the principles of sound learning of which we now take cognisance.

In addition we must appreciate that, as important as the knowledge given at the appropriate stages in development, is the manner in which the knowledge is given, the attitudes and values which are passed on explicitly or conveyed by implication by the personal quality of the teacher and the general ethos of the school itself. We realise it is important that we ensure that, as knowledge and understanding increase, there is also a growing awareness of those values and attitudes which we wish to associate with human sexuality and which we believe should be preserved and passed on.

The aims are positive ones with a lessening of the oppressive and restrictive overtones of earlier years. Our aims for the individual are the promotion of personal maturity, happiness and fulfilment without exploitation of another person. Perhaps a helpful definition of maturity here is that of Ernest Jones, Freud's biographer:

> A mature person is one who is able to give affection in excess of the need to receive it.

and Mrs. Kelmer Pringle's definition of social maturity is also relevant:

> Social maturity is manifest by the extent to which an individual is able and willing to conform to the customs, habits, standards of behaviour and modes prevailing in the society in which he lives by the degree to which he is able to

do so independently of direction and guidance; and by the extent to which he participates constructively in the affairs and conduct of his community.

Child Guidance Inter-Clinic Conference 1963,
National Association of Mental Health

Extensions to the curriculum are taking place at secondary level in many ways including work in Nuffield Science and the Schools Council Projects in Humanities, General Studies and Moral Education, among others. At primary level too the new approaches can include learning which meets the needs and interests of young children in these years from five to eleven or twelve, while at the same time providing the surest foundation for further learning in human sexuality at secondary level and throughout life.

Sex education is part of the totality of learning in the primary school. It is not a separate subject, divorced from other fields of interest. It is part of the wholeness of learning 'the seamless garment of knowledge'. It is also, for each individual child, knowledge which he seeks as an integral part of the drive to come to terms with the real world and to develop a personal identity.

It is the writer's aim to try to help teachers and parents to consider the value to children when they grow up able to learn about themselves and other human beings gradually, as they learn about all other aspects of the real world in schools and homes which give them sufficient security and where the human relationships support them. Then conversation and learning take place on a reciprocal basis, influenced by the interests of the children themselves and guided by teachers who understand them.

Acknowledgements

Many people have had a part in the writing of this book. Its beginnings go back more than twenty years to the boys and girls of South Park Junior School who were the first to show me their interest in their origins and birth.

More recently I have been in less direct contact with children in schools and I am indebted to many of my colleagues, the teachers in and heads of schools in my Authority who have generously shared with me their ideas and experiences of working with children in this sphere of learning, for allowing me to use their own accounts and/or examples or photographs of children's work. I am particularly indebted to:

Miss Pat A. Ballen, Headmistress, Polehampton Infant School.

Mr. Howard Biggs, Headmaster, Childrey County School.

Miss M. E. Cory, Headmistress, Ascot Heath C. E. Junior School.

Mr. C. Cunningham-Burley, Headmaster, Wescott Road County School.

Mr. Geoff Davies, Headmaster, Parsons Down County School.

Mr. Frank Denzey, Headmaster, Chilton County School.
Mr. R. A. Fowler, Headmaster, Grove Junior School.
Mr. R. Free, Ex-Deputy, New Scotland Hill School.
Miss Sue Humphries, Headmistress, The Coombes County Infant School.
Mr. David A. Killick, Headmaster, North Hinksey C. E. School.
Mrs. Mavis Lait, Headmistress, Watchfield County School.
Mrs. Margaret Langford, Deputy Head, Charlton County School.
Mr. D. Lewis, Headmaster, St. Luke's C.E. School.
Miss E. M. Miles, Headmistress, Carswell County Infant School.
Mr. G. W. Taylor, Headmaster, Caldecott County Junior School.
Mr. Paul Vincent, Uffington C. E. School.
Mr. Brian Watkins, Headmaster, Inkpen County School.
Mrs. Renee Westerman, Headmistress, Caldecott County Infant School.
Mrs. E. M. Williams, Headmistress, College Town Infant School.

My thanks too to my colleagues Joan Dean and Frank Poller and to Terry John, Training Officer of the National Marriage Guidance Council, for comments on the final draft and to the Schools' Broadcasting Council of the BBC for permission to quote from their Teachers' booklets.

Lastly one is aware that the development of this work in schools has been possible because of the understanding and support given by my Education Committee and by my Director of Education.

Chapter 1

The ethos of primary/middle schools and conditions for learning about sex

> The foundation for good sexual ethics can be laid in a school in which the children learn to respect and appreciate each other as personalities, to treat everyone with consideration and never make use of human beings or treat them callously or contemptuously and where they find in adults the same attitude towards each other and towards themselves.
>
> *Children and their Primary Schools.* The Plowden Report, 1967.

Primary and first and middle schools are, or are fast becoming, very different from the schools most of us adults remember. Many parents bringing their five-year-olds to school for the first time are surprised and, sometimes, disconcerted by the differences. They hear a busy hum and see a variety of purposeful activities pursued by groups and individuals without a teacher appearing to direct any of them. It may appear to some that the changes have come rapidly, and in some areas they have, but the beginnings of change go back a long way, at least to the early years of the century. They have largely arisen from a clearer picture of childhood derived from many sources, including particularly psychology, anthropology and sociology. This has changed our attitudes to children, the ways in which we organise learning for them and the atmosphere, climate or ethos we try to create in schools so that they are places where children want to be.

The ethos of school is mediated to children through the quality of human relationships between all the people who make up the school community. In a school where relationships enable a child to experience what it is like to receive care, concern and consideration, be respected as an individual, be tolerated, even when feeling anti-social, yet treated consistently and with firmness, when attitudes on the whole seem to be fair and just, he is likely to incorporate these values into himself, almost through the pores of the skin. They will be caught rather than taught. Later in adolescence, when the ability to think in abstractions is usually developed, moral and aesthetic aspects will be added to his personal experience and theoretical knowledge and extend his concept of humanity and human behaviour further. The adolescent boy who does not know what it feels like to be respected will hardly know what the phrase, 'To respect a girl', means. It will be much more difficult to understand the meaning of care and consideration for another person if there has been inadequate first-hand experience in the early years when emotional factors in learning through feelings are very strong.

Similarly, the child who feels loved by mother and father learns to give love by receiving it. The example of adequate love and tolerance between parents affords a constructive model on which their child can begin to build himself. It is significant that a child from a sufficiently happy and loving home nearly always creates such a home in his turn and the child who feels rejected and undervalued often finds it difficult not to be rejecting in adult life.

Sexual love is compounded of all earlier loves, including the love between parent and child, some teachers and child, child and child, including the 'crushes' and hero worship of adolescence. For most of us the closest of all human relationships involves a sexual relationship and it incorporates all the meaningful relationships which each one of us has had from the beginning of life. This means that the personal experience of human relationships of all kinds, even those of the early years in the home and in school, are important for they stay with us all our days and contribute to our degree of maturity as adults.

But for those first affections,
Those shadowy recollections,
Which, be they what they may,
Are yet the fountain-light of all our day,
Are yet a master-light of all our seeing.

William Wordsworth

The first factor for us, as educationists, to consider is therefore the quality of life and learning which permeates a school and creates its particular ethos or atmosphere. It will lie in the personalities of the head and his teachers, the values which generally influence them most and the concept they hold of childhood which together will influence the quality of the relationships in all the activities of ordinary everyday school life. This is probably most readily achieved when a head has a clear concept of standards, both of effort and attainment in an academic sense and of daily conduct in a sense of moral values. When he is able to appoint to his staff teachers who, on the whole, share his aims and ideals and are able to make a positive contribution in their own ways there is a harmony in the school and a shared sense of community.

When the prevailing atmosphere of home and school is sympathetic to children's growing awareness and supports emotional learning through feelings as well as cognitive learning through reasoning, sex education has a place because it is an area of learning concerned both with feelings and with facts. Much of our early learning is through our feelings and we have rudimentary sexual feelings in babyhood. Each one of us acquires, therefore, very early in our lives, an awareness of sex, a hazy picture, a kind of half knowledge through our feelings. Feelings, perhaps engendered by a new baby, kittens, puppies or another child, arouse curiosity and as early as three years of age questions connected with sex begin to be asked. Whether or not questions and talk continue is very dependent on the reaction to the first question or comment. It is usually mother or mother substitute to whom conversation is first addressed and, if the reaction is one of acceptance, and the answer given with ease, then learning will take place and in the child's own time further conversations will follow.

If, however, reaction was one of surprise or tension or anxiety, then the child, who is sensitive to feelings, will withdraw and further conversation will be unlikely to take place because most normal children will avoid creating anxiety.

Professor Jean Piaget has recorded these observations which illustrate clearly this early awareness of sex.

> At 3.3. (28). Y said of her doll Nicholas, 'When he was born he stayed for a long time inside me; he had sharp pointed teeth and afterwards they became smooth.'
>
> At 3.6. (2). she pretended that her son Nicholas's head was in her head, etc.
>
> At 3.9. (13). someone was arguing with her; 'No, don't do that. You know I have a little baby inside me and it hurts him.' Then when the person had gone; 'You know, when my little baby is born, he'll kick him and knock him down.'
>
> At 3.10. (17). she explained to her doll which wanted to be inside her again: 'No, you're too big now, you can't.'
>
> In contrast to this:
>
> At 3.10. (24). Y who wanted to become a boy said to her father: 'I want to go back inside you, and when I come out I'll be a little baby again. I'll be called Y (the masculine form of her name) because I'll be a boy.'*

The second important factor for us to consider, then, is the ability and willingness of teachers to answer children's questions with calm acceptance and serenity in terms the child will understand. As much detail or information as the child wants must be given but, at the same time, it must be borne in mind that often a short to-the-point answer is what is wanted and that where attitudes are supporting the child, supplementary questions will be put if more information is wanted.

It is also important to realise that an acceptable and satisfying answer must be given as soon as possible or be found in books, etc. by teacher and child or parent and child together, for we know that the ability to frame a question reveals partial knowledge of what the answer will be, a real desire to know more and a certain trust in the adult's ability to help in this. To fob a child off with a partial answer or to be evasive is to discourage learning in general; to fob a child off when the question is closely tied to

---

*Jean Piaget, *Play, Dreams and Imitation in Childhood*. New York, Norton, 1951. pp. 173–4.

personal development seems now, in the light of present knowledge, to be irresponsible.

In the sort of school being described here children are likely to feel able to ask any questions, even those which, in the actual asking, they know could seem to others rather silly and idiosyncratic. They will expect their teachers to treat their queries with sympathy and trust them to give an accurate answer or help them to find the information they want. Muddles and confusions of sexual matters are very common and some children need to unlearn a muddle before they can come to an accurate understanding at the level appropriate to their ability.

Teachers who fully understand children are most likely to realise that some children have learned long before they come into school that there is an area of life, facts about part of their own bodies, observable aspects of themselves and others, about which they must not seek information. They have learned not to ask questions. To meet this situation it is important that the teacher accepts the responsibility for initiating learning by organising the learning environment and school day so that she makes this area appropriate and relevant to the learning in general and therefore makes it easy for children to talk about sexuality, babies and animal babies, etc. and ask questions. On the other hand it is no more important to initiate learning here than in mathematics, or reading, or formation of letters for writing, but it is *as* important and the aim should be to engineer the learning with skill, sensitivity and balance and to make it relevant and appropriate for the child, so that it is part of the whole learning and integrated into whatever aspect of the curriculum is appropriate.

Teachers with years of experience and possessing real teaching skill have said that they have never been asked questions on babies, birth or any aspect of sex by a child in school. This is understandable. Older teachers, like many other people of their generation, have not been accustomed to talk about subjects connected with sex in their private life, and in their professional training this part of learning for young children would not have been mentioned because the need to include it in the curriculum was not appreciated. This is true of many other areas of the curriculum which we now make available to children in schools. The primary school curriculum is expanding all the time and embraces more areas of learning today than ever before.

This means that such a teacher's attitude, while supporting children in many ways, will not make it easy for children to talk or ask questions about everything. Children are sensitive to feelings and will sense that to question such a teacher about certain topics will make the teacher anxious and this they will always avoid doing. If the teacher is also regarded with affection, as are most teachers of young children, they are even more unlikely to be asked questions or to be included in a conversation which the children sense will worry them.

Learning about sex has started long before children come into school and the school must take account of this. A third factor to consider therefore is whether one's particular school is joining or has joined the increasing number of schools which have taken note of the Plowden recommendations and research, on home and school relationships, and actively pursue a policy to promote partnership between parents and teachers in the education of the child. Such schools are likely to be ones which note the home circumstances from which the child comes each morning and to which he returns each night. They will also recognise that education takes place twenty-four hours out of twenty-four in the interactions between the child and all persons who impinge upon his consciousness and that his teacher is only one of many people who influence him. For the further learning to be relevant and meaningful the teacher must be able to accept what the child already knows and lead him on from it. Partnership between parents and teachers is important in all learning if a child is to achieve his full potential. In sex education this co-operation and understanding is particularly valuable for, as will be explained further later on, an element in sex education for young children is discovery of self and only the parents can supplement the teacher's work by giving the child data on his own background, birth, babyhood and development to enable him to build up an integrated picture of himself.

For schools which serve areas of social and economic deprivation and receive children from homes which are less educationally supporting than we would wish, a fourth factor needs to be considered. This is that in these schools it is likely that the teachers will not have the same degree of co-operation from parents in sex education as schools which serve more favoured areas. This is because it could be difficult for many of these parents to understand the child's need for knowledge or how to give it if they did. This will come in time, as the views of more educated and enlightened parents gradually percolate to them. For the present, however, schools in most poor areas will need to compensate children for inadequate learning at home and accept responsibility for leading the child to a gradual understanding of the facts and an awareness of values and attitudes to sex which may be contrary to those acquired in the home. It is, as teachers experienced in these schools will know, important never to imply criticism of the child's background. In sex education this is particularly important for quite young children in infant schools have sometimes already been severely hurt by prevailing sexual *mores* and are sensitive to criticism. The school's aim, through the individual teacher's approach, can be one of offering, over the years, an alternative picture of human behaviour and family life for the child to carry inside him, so that in adolescence he may recall the experience gained in school to set up alongside that of his home and perhaps choose to be influenced in his adult behaviour more by his school than by his home.

The fifth and last factor for us to bear in mind is one of organisation for learning which affords opportunities for the child to talk to the teacher on his own. This is common in more and more schools where there is recognition of the importance of noting the individuality of each child and his established mode of growth and pattern of learning. In such schools most teachers will observe the way in which each child behaves and learns and will arrange the provision, the task or activity so that learning is efficient and economic for that child. Learning will still be by direct teaching, when this is most profitable, but is less likely to be with a whole class and more often with groups and individuals than in the past. This gives greater opportunity for conversation on a one-to-one basis which is the most effective form of communication and also enables the child to ask questions and talk about matters of personal and, at times, private interest if he wishes.

The atmosphere or ethos of a school, though easy to recognise, is difficult to define. It is not amenable to measurement or assessment and yet it is the most potent influence. It outlasts the facts learned, games played and activities enjoyed and yet these are also part of it.

Ethos is derived from persons, and in schools these will be

children, head, teachers, secretary, cook, auxiliaries and care-taker—in fact all who make up a school community. In primary, or first and middle, schools in particular the ethos will stem from the beliefs and personal qualities of the head. When the atmosphere is right for children they tend themselves to con-tribute to it by their behaviour and hence support it.

There are a few features one can pick out as common in schools with a child-centred atmosphere but these are just a few and they are each an aspect of human relationships. Usually there are a sufficient number of teachers who can stimulate learning and at the same time preserve a calm serenity. They can be busy and hard working and yet have time for the individual. They can accept even the seemingly difficult and unlikable and yet convey likable qualities which a child might constructively incorporate into himself. They can be accepting of the individual without necessarily condoning his behaviour. They belong to the com-munity to which they contribute and in a sense also receive some-thing from it themselves. There is a mutual giving and receiving at all levels from the oldest to the youngest. Relationships are symbiotic and conducive to individual development and the achievement of happiness and well-being without exploitation of another person or persons.

Perhaps this can be summed up by saying that a school com-munity with such an ethos which supports children is composed of a sufficient number of adults who care. They care about emotional development and mental health, they care about standards, performance and the quality of learning, and they care about the aesthetic and moral influences which in these years are conveyed to children by the examples of adults in ordinary day-to-day living and only a little by precept and rules which have little meaning for children at this age.

As this chapter started with a quotation from the Plowden Report, perhaps it is helpful to end with one which puts in another way some of the ideas on ethos or atmosphere of schools which one is attempting to convey.

A school is not merely a teaching shop, it must transmit values and attitudes. It is a community in which children learn to live first and foremost as children and not as future adults. In family life children learn to live with people of all ages. The school sets out deliberately to devise the right environment for children, to allow them to be themselves and to develop in the way and at the pace appropriate to them. It tries to equalise opportunities and to compensate for handicaps. It lays special stress on individual discovery, on first-hand experience and on opportunities for creative work. It insists that knowledge does not fall into neatly separate compartments and that work and play are not opposite but complementary. A child brought up in such an atmosphere at all stages of his education has some hope of becoming a balanced and mature adult and of being able to live in, to contribute to and to look critically at the society of which he forms a part.

Chapter 2

The meaning of sex education in the early years and its contribution to development

This book is intended for adult reading. The term 'sex education' is deliberately being used so that the area of learning under discussion is clearly defined for the adults concerned. It is the term explicity used in the Plowden Report, *Children and Their Primary Schools,* and was used by the British Broadcasting Corporation in their Further Education Programme for teachers and parents. Most headmasters and headmistresses have been equally explicit and straightforward in their letters to parents inviting them for talks and discussions on the subject.

When, however, we in schools, and in homes, are concerned with children themselves we are most unlikely to use the words sex education or sex because the sexual relationships conveyed to adults by these words are irrelevant to the interests and under-standing of children in the early years.

For pre-school, infant and junior school children this know-ledge is viewed much more as a part of self-discovery, being a story about me, all about my baby brother or baby sister or the baby next door, all about us, my family, families, human beings. The sexual aspect, including intercourse, tends on the whole to be regarded as an action which starts off a sequence of events or a story and it is the main body of the story which is of most interest, this being how a baby grows before it is born and how it is born. Most children identify themselves with the baby and it is the centre of their interest in the cognitive sense of learning facts and at the same time in the emotional sense of eliciting warm feelings, often of protection towards a smaller version of themselves (see Fig. 1). Children often express in their different ways a marked sense of satisfaction when they know that a baby, including they themselves, grows or grew inside the mother. In schools their painting, drawing and writing often reveal this (see Figs. 2 and 3). It contributes to a sense of security. It seems to be information which is absolutely right for that period of development when the child likes being cuddled, nestling upon a comforting lap and being held securely.

Children's recordings in writing and art, their conversation in a secure environment, their free drama and play, and behaviour in other ways, suggest that there can be a psychological gain to the individual who learns bit by bit about his origins while he is

Figure 1

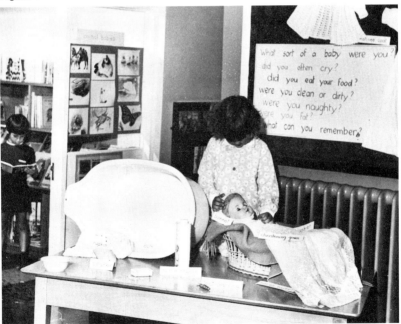

Figure 2

Figure 3

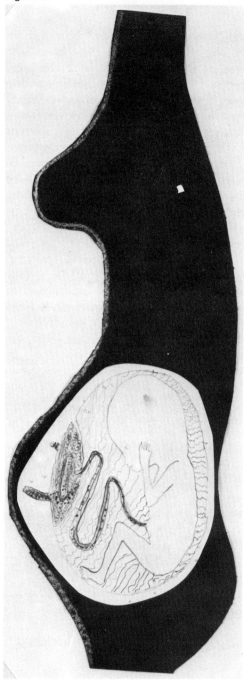

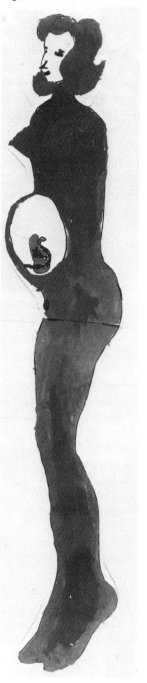

still near enough to his own babyhood to identify with the baby, imagine he is a baby again and possibly experience what can be simply described as an imaginative rebirth. It allows understanding to grow gradually in line with development and thus from many different standpoints. While learning in the early years, with an imaginative step backwards to identification with the baby, probably assists the acquisition of self-awareness; in learning, in the years of adolescence, the majority of girls and boys will no longer associate with the baby but imaginatively project themselves forward to the adult sexual roles they will play. In this anticipation of future roles learning may involve an increase in factual knowledge and it can also be a preparation for adult life and its responsibilities if education provides for it.

Knowledge that a baby is made from the sperm of the father and the ovum of the mother, and the feeling within the child that he is of both his father and his mother make a gradual and positive contribution to the child's understanding of himself (see Figs. 4 and 5). In everything in which he is involved, in his interaction with people, all the activities of home and school, and in all the learning, reading, writing and mathematics, etc., of these years the child is building up a clearer and clearer vision of himself and achieving an increasing measure of integration of personality. He gradually acquires the ability to behave with greater consistency according to the character or personality he is becoming. Around seven or eight years of age a child needs his parents and teachers to confirm, by their behaviour towards him, that he is the sort of person he believes himself to be. He needs his internal picture of himself, his idea of his identity, to be confirmed by those adults whom he trusts. Simple facts which link all children to their parents and through them to their grandparents, etc. contribute to the individual child's sense of belonging. It gives him a clearer idea of his place in the family, extended family, and neighbourhood. It helps him to understand his physical characteristics, why he is shorter or taller than his friend, a bit like his father and with a particular feature of his mother's. It gives factual information to complement the unique individual phantasy picture he has of himself which he has learned chiefly through his feelings. Understanding of facts fills out the rather hazy picture, removes the feeling of inadequacy and eliminates the questioning feelings which arise from knowing one has only partial knowledge, and hence contributes to integration of

Figure 4

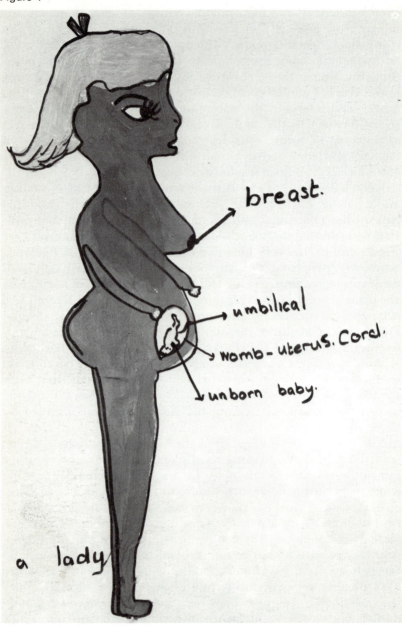

breast.

umbilical

womb - uterus. Cord.

unborn baby.

a lady

Figure 5

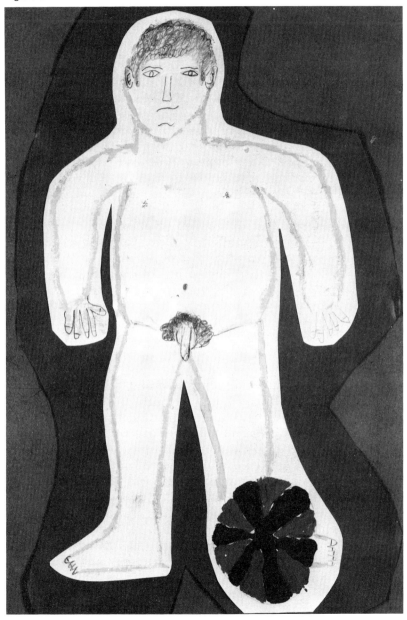

personality, sense of identity and confidence. Such knowledge establishes a fundamental basis for a growing understanding of the common bond of humanity, that all of us come into the world in the same way and yet that each is unique. It is information which makes sense of our feelings and fulfils the child's desire for order. Confidence derived from such knowledge helps the child to move forward with ease into learning in all areas of a curriculum.

In addition to the development of a sense of identity or of an integrated personality, the primary school years are also concerned with acquiring the ability to cope with anxiety. Anxiety is endemic to the human condition and a factor with which we all have to cope throughout life. It is an aspect of mental health. It is also an element in motivation to learning. Perhaps in this context it is more readily understood when viewed as Piaget's disequilibrium which can be described as a feeling which we have when we are faced with the unfamiliar, or a new aspect of a situation, or a problem which we cannot immediately solve. Learning takes place when we take positive action to control the situation by thinking and thus by coming to a degree of understanding regain an equilibrium.

Anxiety is necessary for learning and survival, while a factor in mental health is the degree of anxiety which an individual can tolerate. It is rather like the shaving-stick advertisement; we want 'Not too little, not too much, but just right'. The gradual acquisition of the degree which is 'just right' is made in all the activities in which the child is involved and will be most easily made when the adults create a secure environment and present challenges to thinking which are on the whole appropriate to the individual's ability to cope but are nevertheless adequately challenging.

Anxiety is built up when the child is confronted too often with things over which he cannot gain a degree of understanding and control which affords him satisfaction. We know that withholding information when curiosity is aroused can create anxiety in some children. When curiosity is evoked even by ordinary everyday observable things like babies, pregnancy and overt sexual behaviour, anxiety can be reinforced over and over again. For those who live in less favoured conditions such as some crowded homes, or with unstable parents or where there is a changing series of men each playing the role of father, etc., acute anxiety can be created by confusion caused by witnessing adult behaviour which more responsible parents, or parents better housed, would not allow their children to see. Because there is strong motivation, or a driving urge, in young children to find an answer to problems and satisfy curiosity, what they cannot answer from fact they will answer by phantasy. Phantasy solutions, however, rely solely on feelings which fluctuate and change and can therefore never be satisfactory. When accurate knowledge is withheld for too long some children's phantasy solutions become over-fixed, they get tangled up in it, and then, when it is possible for them to learn accurately what is fact and reality, it can be difficult for them. They have too much unlearning to do before they can learn. They also find it harder to trust an adult when their experience has been of evasiveness, which has contributed to anxiety. Underlying anxiety about one part of learning or one area of the curriculum can effect learning in all other areas. Anxiety holds a child back, it prevents an embracing, on-going approach to new ideas and thinking. It militates against learning.

Concepts develop in complexity throughout life. In the pre-school nursery or infant school years most learning is through perception and practical first-hand experience. Gradually, however, there is a need for more and more relevant theory to amplify the knowledge gained through practical situations to combine with self-discovery and reasoning at both practical and abstract levels. The primary school is concerned with the early stages of theoretical learning—the introduction to, or foundations for, more subject-based learning in secondary schools.

In the area of learning we have defined it is necessary for children to learn theory which is relevant to their interest, curiosity and understanding at different times and this will provide a foundation for more detailed knowledge at later stages. It is important that this foundation is well laid and for this to be so we must ensure that it is adequately detailed for the child's need and accurate so that there is no need for correction at later stages. An important element in accuracy is the acquisition of an adequate vocabulary of acceptable words and in this case of scientific terminology.

Possibly, because of the influence of personal feelings which are always associated with parts of the body, there is a tendency for different kinds of in-language to exist. Some families have

17

their own 'baby' names for the external genitalia and so on. It is important that, when the child comes to school, he should gradually acquire the accurate terms to set beside his personal family ones. Accurate language is likely to take over as learning proceeds in the terms defined by language itself.

Acquisition of language is indissolubly linked with thinking and reasoning, and with feelings too. There will be no meaningful acquisition of vocabulary if at the time a word is given there is not also ample and relevant opportunity for the word to be used. Home and school must accept that if a word has meaning for a child and it is relevant to his thinking he will need to use it to communicate his ideas and at the same time clarify them. Therefore parents and teachers will need to create situations where it is easy, comfortable and opportune to do this. In homes where there is sympathy for children this will happen in the course of daily life—the odd comment over the egg for breakfast or the roes in the herring for supper and, more frequently perhaps, at bath time or bed time. In schools, too, conversation directly concerned with this topic, and related to it in different ways, will take place in all sorts of situations including mathematics, news time, in stories and in play, provided the teacher's attitude is sufficiently supporting. This will be largely determined by his or her acceptance of the relevance of this area of learning to the children in the class or learning group.

In this area, as in most learning, nouns are likely to be acquired first; for in the acquisition of the correct name there is the definition of terms essential for learning to take place. The practical aspect, the function of the noun, brings in verbs and then adverbs and adjectives for description and comparison at different times for different children. Those parts of the body which the child observes most readily are likely to be named and explained first and most children, except the least able, will learn this in supporting homes before entry to school. It is worth remembering, however, that there is much evidence to show that children from linguistically deprived backgrounds enter school with fewer nouns and in this context will not know less obvious parts of the body such as elbow, wrist, penis and breast, etc. In the learning of theory there is the acquisition of more and more precise language, and the interaction of learning and precise language leads to greater accuracy and understanding.

While it is important for homes and schools to provide appropriate opportunities to talk about this subject, it is equally important for children to learn as they grow older when it is inappropriate to talk about it, that not all situations are suitable places for conversation on personal matters. They will need to learn that not all people find frank discussion on this subject acceptable and that in some circumstances to hold such a conversation is bad manners and inconsiderate to the feelings of others. They will gradually learn that the subject is one which is concerned largely with private and personal affairs, and the majority will acquire a certain reticence according to their personality which most of us would feel to be desirable. Reticence involves an awareness of the feelings of others as well as oneself and is not the same thing as inhibition, which is to be overwhelmed by inner feelings which can be emotionally retarding.

Suggestions on vocabulary details and ways of introducing learning about babies of all kinds, families, etc. are given in the next chapters on curriculum. What one would like to stress here is that the approach is not new. It is good infant/junior-primary school practice. The only new element is that it is an extension of the curriculum and dependent entirely on the teacher's willingness to allow the extension to take place. This will develop very much on children's terms once they know that learning about themselves and others is included and not, as before, excluded from discussion in schools. Many teachers who have incorporated this into the integrated learning programme or into more subject-based curricula have said that they do not know now why they prevaricated or what difficulties they had really anticipated—that any difficulty was in themselves and that for the children the subject was so relevant that their interest shaped the approach and organisation and the amount of learning undertaken.

Chapter 3

Curriculum for the early years: five to eight

It is likely that the inclusion of appropriate learning in the infant school or first school is more dependent on the attitude of the teacher to sex education than it is at any later stages. This is because the best approach seems, on the whole, to be when this learning is incidental to and part of the whole learning process. If the teacher believes that this is an aspect of the real world, the child's environment in which he is interested and requires information, she will be aware of the opportunities which occur for learning to take place easily and naturally, yet purposefully, in innumerable ways; in the contexts of, for instance, mathematics, science, exploration of home and school environment, stories, poems, drama, communication of all kinds and in religious education. She will, when it is necessary, sensitively 'open the door' on this area of learning by introducing it in an appropriate way or by planning situations in which it is easy for children to learn if they are interested.

The following accounts given by the headmistress of an infant school which receives many children of Air Force personnel, who, therefore, move frequently from school to school, reflects this sensitive, purposeful approach:

All the work we do is incidental.

We endeavour to make children aware of the family unit: the different roles played by father and mother, their own place in the family, etc.

With children constantly coming and going, the children are continually aware of the needs of a newcomer and they are always ready to make any newcomer feel welcome by showing the whereabouts of toilets, cloakroom, dining halls, etc. Children travelling on buses know that new people need someone to show them bus stops, etc., and so will volunteer to stay with them until they become able to cope on their own. The older children in particular are protective towards new entrants.

The teachers give the children opportunities to ask questions, they give openings for discussions and they will take up observations, etc., so that they can be enlarged to the extent the children wish to take them. Lengthy discussions are not forced on them. In this sort of atmosphere where the children are free to talk to the teacher in a small group situation they will often answer one another's questions, appealing to the teacher when they feel the need for extra information or affirmation of their own statements as in these examples:

A child came into school and said he had seen a hedgehog.

Child: 'Do mother hedgehogs lay eggs so that they can have baby hedgehogs?'

Teacher: 'No, baby hedgehogs grow in their mummies' tummies like you did.'

Child: 'Did I really grow in my mummy's tummy?'

Teacher: 'Yes, you did.'

Child: 'Well, if a baby grows in its mummy's tummy, how does it know when to come out?'

Teacher: 'It knows it must stay there until it is big and strong.'

Child: 'How does the baby come out? Does it have to make a hole?'

Teacher: 'No, the hole is already there.'

There was a small pause. One or two looked somewhat mystified, as though they might be trying to form a question and then suddenly started talking about something different.

The teacher allowed the discussion to close. Most of the children in this group were boys 4+ to 5+ years.

A group of children 6+ to 7+ years were planting seeds. They were talking with the teacher about the seeds and their size; how tiny they were and what they would grow into, etc. Gradually the conversation progressed until the teacher said: 'You were very, very tiny before you grew into a baby in your mummy's tummy'.

A gruff voice in an undertone from Richard (newly arrived from Australia). 'Not true, not true.'

Teacher: 'What makes you think I am not telling you the truth?'

Richard: 'Well, I know it's not true. It can't be. I came from Australia, I know I did, so I know I did not grow in my mummy's tummy'.

This rejection from Richard was definite and explosive. He just could not accept what was said. The other children ignored the statement and continued with what they were doing. The teacher felt that no good purpose could be achieved by pressing the point.

Some time later I overheard this conversation between Richard and John, as they were painting in the cloakroom.

John: 'Oh, look, it is raining.'

Richard: 'Raining, it mustn't be, it can't be.'

John: 'Why, what is wrong because it is raining?'

Richard: 'Well, I don't want it to rain this afternoon. The lady next door has a baby in her tummy. It's hurting her quite a lot so she wants to go to hospital this afternoon and have it taken out, so I don't want it to rain. I want it to be nice for her.'

I felt that Richard had come to terms with the fact and was pleased with his attitude to the woman concerned.

A child brought a book to school which had a picture on the cover of a stork carrying a baby.

Conversation between the children:

Question: What is that bird?

Answer: A stork.

Question: What is he carrying?

Answer: A baby.

Question: Why is it carrying a baby?
Answer: Because storks bring babies.
Comment: Of course the stork doesn't bring babies. Babies grow in the mummy's tummy, don't they, Mrs. S.?
Teacher: Yes, that's right.
Question: Then if the stork does not bring babies why do people say it does?
Teacher: Because that is a make-up story. People love storks and people love babies, so some people made up the story that storks bring babies. You know we have true stories and make-up stories: the story of the stork is a make-up story, but when we say a baby grows in its mummy's tummy, that is true.

Clare and Mary were sitting together looking through a book of pictures. (Reproductions of Old Masters.) As they were turning the pages they came across a picture in which a nude woman was depicted. Mary looked at Clare, pointed to the figure and gave a little giggle. Clare looking very serious: 'Why are you laughing?' Mary still pointed to the figure but looked surprised at Clare's reaction, as it was obvious Mary would have liked a little giggle. Clare: 'What is there to laugh at? I can't see anything to laugh at, are you laughing because you think it's rude? It isn't rude, you know, it's not rude at all. Anyway we shall look like that another day.' As far as Clare was concerned the matter was finished, so she turned the page to look at the next picture.

For most children early learning interest is likely to be of short duration requiring a small item of information at a time, perhaps a confirmation of a child's own statement: for example, Boys and girls are different between the legs, aren't they?' One suggests that the answer required here may be no more than Yes, they are', and that the teacher conveys a willingness to discuss the subject further if the child wishes. She may ask a question 'Do you know how they are different?' and go on from here. No one can teach a teacher how to convey this sort of attitude or 'openness' with sensitivity. It is part of a general attitude to children but there are certainly very many who, from the beginning of their careers, have this skill and many others who acquire it, as part of their own development, as teachers.

The degree of interest will vary here as in all fields of learning. It is likely to be very strong at times and, when a degree of knowledge is sufficient for the time being, there are likely to follow periods when the subject will be rarely mentioned.

One would not wish to advocate any one particular curriculum or any one particular approach, for the socio-economic background of the children will vary from school to school and within any one school. The degree of knowledge with which children enter school will vary, also its accuracy and the ways in which it was acquired. Teachers vary too, in the ways in which they work with children, and should feel free to adopt the approaches with which they themselves feel secure. This is particularly true when the area is new to the curriculum. These factors, and possibly others, will need to be taken into account in planning the content of the curriculum and the best approaches to use. Although it is important, in planning curricula, for each teacher to do her own thinking and plan content and method to suit her own circumstances, one is aware that many teachers would be glad of some help with this. The following suggestions are put forward as guide-lines only and they are followed by a selection of some approaches used successfully by different teachers in different kinds of schools.

Curriculum

This is factual knowledge which is relevant to most children's interests and assists all-round development in these years. Children will have opportunities in the active infant school or first school to learn these facts bit by bit, incidentally, by about seven or eight years of age, depending on the individual child and its relevance to interest. Nothing here is beyond the interest and early understanding of this age group any more than initial learning about fractions, as far as understanding allows, is beyond infant school children.

The items of information can be listed under the following title:

Where Babies Come From. Human babies and some animal babies (Mammals).
Babies grow inside their mothers.

Babies grow from a tiny ovum about as big as a pencil dot, or a grain of salt, or . . .

They are born through the vagina.

The baby is born alive and can cry and kick and wave his arms.

He is about twenty-one inches long when he is born.

Baby feeds on milk from mother's breast or from a bottle.

Babies soon begin to look a little bit like their parents, because . . .

Babies are made from part of the father (sperm) and part of the mother (ovum).

Babies of different kinds (humans compared with animals) take different lengths of time to grow up.

Human babies take the longest time of all to grow up.

Human babies have a lot to learn before they are toddlers;

toddlers before they are ready to be schoolboys and girls;

schoolboys and girls before they are adolescents, and teenagers before they are grown up.

It helps to have a mother and a father in a home to grow up with.

Most human beings, but not all, live in families of different sizes.

Babies are born either girl babies (female) or boy babies (male).

There are differences between boys (males) and girls (females), men (males) and women (females).

The chief difference between boys and girls is between the legs.

Boys have a penis and girls have labia with a vagina.

These differences are the same for all boys and girls; all men and women, of all colours and races.

We can often tell when a woman is pregnant.

Doctors and nurses often help a mother when a baby is born.

Some babies are born in hospitals or maternity homes and some in their homes.

It is suggested that these facts which children like to know should be learned incidentally where appropriate and hence some will learn some facts first and some will learn others first. Therefore there can be no definite order laid down for this. Nevertheless the above reflects a fairly common order in children's thinking in a very general way.

Vocabulary

It is suggested that the following words should be used whenever appropriate. Again the child's ability to use these words easily and naturally will depend on understanding, but at the same time the correct terminology will assist in the clarification of terms and classification which promotes understanding. Different children will acquire vocabulary in different order and it is likely to be related to the order in which they gain understanding of the theory.

Words for parts of the body

All of these words are terms for external parts of the body and therefore observable by the child. He will discover them for himself but he will be dependent on an adult to name them for him:

Head	chest	abdomen	limb
hair—on the head,—chest—under-arm,		pubic hair	
breast	nipple	bosom	
abdomen	navel		
anus	buttock		
penis	scrotum	labia	vagina

Other parts of the body not connected with this particular area of knowledge will of course be learned when relevant, for this will obviously help to keep a balanced approach.

Additional words relevant to the subject

pregnant	reproduce	reproduction	maternity	midwife
male	sperm	female	ovum	uterus
birth	born			
urine	urinate	urination		
faeces	defecate	defecation		
mammal	milk	suck	wean	

The clear definition of urination and defecation is helpful for young children. It can contribute to their development when a teacher is able to allow children to learn accurately and check up on their own ideas on these two functions. They are more emotionally pleasurable functions for children than they become in later life and muddled ideas about sex can start from confusion between anus and vagina. A not insignificant number of children, learning largely through their feelings, believe that a baby is born through the anus and sometimes acquire emotional associations of defecation with sexuality which may continue to affect their development into adolescence and adult life.

Learning can take place in all sorts of contexts:

Storytime is the easiest approach for some teachers, for story reading is a part of the school day in which all infant teachers have some experience. It allows an oblique approach which is sometimes wise if it is the initial introduction and the teacher will judge whether the children identify with the story or whether she will need to help with this by drawing parallels between the children's life and the story situation.

The following books are all suitable for reading to children and it is suggested that, after they have been introduced by the teacher, most are put on the children's bookshelves for children to use themselves:

1. *Peter and Caroline*. Stan Hegeler (Tavistock).

A good story-book for infants which the teacher could read to the children in groups and they could later read themselves. Affords opportunity for the teacher to show her willingness to answer children's questions, discuss personal relationships and help the child towards a development of sound attitudes. From such an introduction information on human life and reproduction could continue to be given according to interest and stages of development. A good book to recommend to parents.

2. *How the Baby Came*. Dorotheen Allan and Marie Neurath
(Heinemann).

A family story of Mummy, Daddy, John and Mary and how their new baby brother was born. Well written and clearly illustrated. Reads aloud well for infants and is a good class library book for lower juniors.

Like *Peter and Caroline* the story gives the teacher the opportunity to introduce the subject and show her willingness to discuss personal interests with the children if they wish.

3. *How John Grew an Inch*. D. Allan and M. Neurath
(Heinemann).

Similar to the previous one, concentrating on growing.

4. *How Babies are Made*. A. Andry and S. Schepp
(Time-Life International).

A fairly good book for parents to read with children from about the age of three, for teachers to use with groups of infants and for children to use themselves throughout the primary school. A very simple account which answers all the main questions children are known to ask written with advice from the Child Study Association of America. Illustrations are in paper sculpture and on the whole illustrate the text clearly.

5. *The Wonderful Story of How You Were Born*. S. M. Gruenberg
(World Books).

One of the best books for children to read for themselves. Written with real understanding of young children's development.

6. *Dan Berry's New Baby*. Anthony Jones (Blackie, 1969).

One of four supplementary readers in a series on real life situations: *Life with Dan Berry*. Suitable for reading to younger children and for children of about eight years to read to themselves. All four books could be in the class library.

7. *Animal Babies*. Alice Day Pratt. (Beacon Press, Boston).

The Family Finds Out. Edith Fisher Hunter.
(Beacon Press, Boston).

Always Growing. Elizabeth M. Manwell.
(Beacon Press, Boston).

Martin and Judy. Vol. 1 3–4 Verna Hills Bayley.
Vol. 2 4–5 Verna Hills Bayley.
Vol. 3 5–6 Verna Hills Bayley.

The last six books above set out to meet the needs and to allay the anxieties of young children, which arise in the family and later in school in making personal relationships with adults, siblings, new babies and animals and in understanding life and living in all its aspects. The birth of young animals, the death of a pet, the preparation for and birth of a new baby are included in the family-centred stories. They are exceedingly valuable as examples of a way in which children can be helped to make relationships and acquire attitudes of consideration and concern for others. They have an ethical purpose.

They provide the kind of setting in infant classes in which children's questions can be answered and, more important still, offer the child the opportunity to ask his own questions which he may have suppressed because of adult inhibition or lack of awareness to this need. By the use of these types of stories a parent and/or teacher is able to show the child their willingness to give information on deeply felt aspects of living including human reproduction, but at the same time a balance is preserved so that the information given can be relevant to the child's needs.

The stories are written for American children and the vernacular is unsuitable for children in this country. Infant teachers will, however, find them helpful and language will easily be modified by a good story-teller.

The headmistress of a two-form entry infant school which serves the poorer area of a small historic town finds these books valuable. She says:

> I feel as far as children in the Infant School are concerned our approach to sex education must be in the context of a secure and homely situation where the relationship between teacher and child is one of trust and encourages the child to ask questions as they occur within the environment created in the school to stimulate interest and curiosity. To this end we have also included in our selection for the school library these books, and one teacher reports that individual children looking at these books asked pertinent questions which she answered as they arose.

The New Baby. Taylor and Ingleby (Longman).
What's Inside. May Garelick (The World's Work)
Through the Year. (Author's name not given in book).
   New Colour Photo Book 13 (E. J. Arnold).
The Private Lives of Animals (Frederick Warne).
        (Translated by F. D. Fawcett. Edited by John Clegg).
Let's Read and Find Out Science Books (A. and C. Black).
   Watch Honeybees with Me. Judy Hawes.
   A Tree is a Plant. Clyde Robert Bulla.
Nikolai Lives in Moscow. Deana Levin (Methuen).
Noriko-San—Girl of Japan. Astrid Lindgren (Methuen).
Galahad the Guinea Pig. Anne Marie Pajot (Nelson).
The Big Cats. Desmond Morris (Bodley Head).
The Junior True Book of Horses. Elsa Posell (Frederick Muller).
Animals at Home. Marion Koenig (Chambers).
   The Beaver.
   The Bee.

Exploring the Park. Leslie Jackman (Evans Bros.).
Exploring the Hedgerows. Leslie Jackman (Evans Bros.).
Nature at Home. Elsie Proctor (A. and C. Black).
   Looking at Nature.
Your Body. Ladybird.
Macdonald's First Library Books:
   Cats ⎫
 • *Frogs* ⎪
   Toads ⎬ Chief Editor: Angela Sheehan, B.A.
   Under the Sea ⎭
Pets' Series: I. L. Mackenzie and R. Radford
   Hamsters, Budgerigars, Dogs,   (Basil Blackwell).
   Cats, Mice, Goldfish, Tortoises.

Other new books on this subject are coming on the market now. Teachers are wise to read them through and study the illustrations to ensure that they not only make facts clear, but also contribute to the values the teacher believes should be conveyed. There is a tendency at present for some books to include more explicit illustrative material than seems in our experience necessary for understanding at primary level, e.g. close-up photographs of adult external genitalia and detailed coloured drawings of a cross section showing intercourse. This sort of reference book may occasionally be helpful for a small number of junior school age children of high intellectual ability when they are working for a while closely with the teacher. It will not be relevant to most children's interest. More and more primary schools adopt ways of working with books where the teacher is not necessarily in close contact with the child or group all the time and one would personally hesitate to have this sort of illustration freely available so that a child could come across it when in a particular mood, maybe feeling a little rejected and unappreciated, and in such a mood perhaps find it disturbing.

In newstime or even more likely in the conversation which goes on throughout the day, most infant school children will talk about all sorts of things including the birth of a sibling or neighbour's baby because they are affected or involved. For many years now teachers have talked to children about their new babies and have known that it is helpful when they can share in the pleasure the child may have or show understanding of jealousy or rivalry. It has not, however, necessarily been appreciated that this often provides just the right opportunity gently to find out how much the children know, followed by simple information to supplement what is known already. In any group one child will always know more than another about any topic and conversely one will know least. One of the values of group discussion is that children learn from each other, from teacher's answers to other children's questions, in addition to the answer they receive to their own. Writing about newstime and other similar occasions a headmistress of another infant school writes:

> I feel that a good basic relationship in the beginnings of sex education has been built up between the teachers and the children in this school. All teachers are quite prepared to answer any questions which the children may ask and we feel that the majority of the children at newstime and on other occasions discuss freely the arrival of new babies, kittens, puppies and domestic issues, which affect them through the advent of additions to the family.

In mathematical activities such as weighing and measuring, children often weigh themselves and measure their heights and parts of their own bodies. This is not only assisting understanding of mathematics but making a contribution to an understanding of self. Recordings by the use of different kinds of graphs and diagrams, for instance, can follow. Comparisons may be made and perhaps the tallest boy or girl is discovered, or the shortest. From this could come something like—'Why is John so tall?' 'His father is very tall'. 'He is like his father because John is made from part of his father and part of his mother. (We are all made from part of our father and part of our mother.)' Reference to family likenesses may arise in many other situations—for instance in learning about sets—all the fair-haired in this set, all the dark-haired in that set. Family likeness and relationships will also be observed in different creatures and plants when children are involved in handling animals and keeping and breeding them where this is possible.

> 'Today susannas mummy brout jennys puppies the brown dog was coulde choclate and the black dog was coulde licquerice, the father was brown and so was Jenny.'

'Today sussana's mum came to school with the puppies. They were 2 puppies. I like the 2 puppies and the daddy was older than the mummy dog. They were 25 cm.'

Mathematics involving the weighing of animal babies and keeping a record of their gain in weight would assist in understanding growth. Children might also find out how much they themselves weighed when born, then weigh themselves at school and calculate their gain.

Many other topics which are essentially mathematical can also incorporate learning about oneself. These are, at the same time, a relevant part of sex education.

The environment of the school and its surroundings offer opportunities of many different kinds. A possible one is a study of homes and families; a simple analysis of the different homes in which the children live, for example, houses, bungalows, flats, caravans, or an analysis of family size could be a way of introducing the idea of families and how they are started. Family occasions of weddings and christenings do the same.

Visits to farms and studies of farm life, particularly different types of animal husbandry, obviously offer marvellous opportunities for children to begin to learn about young animals and how they are carried in their mothers and are born and cared for. A head of an infant school reported:

Recently I was talking to a group of children about the young lambs which some of them had seen on a visit to a local farm, and they discussed unreservedly the animal mothers which they knew fed their young. Then one boy said, "Human mothers feed their babies with milk from their breasts."

This freedom to express thoughts, and the children knowing that the adults around are ready and willing to listen and talk about what interests them is, I believe, the right beginning in helping them to acquire knowledge about sex as and when they are ready. We, as teachers, having provided the opportunity to watch and care for animal families in school can help to develop the children's understanding by suggesting books the children can read, and work they can do, in following up their comments and questions.

I do feel it is important that heads of infant schools, such as I, should organise the programme with a view to giving the teachers opportunity to break down the large groups for which they are responsible into smaller new ones occasionally. In this way the teacher has a chance to converse with the children and make helpful discoveries into the way they are thinking.

Visits to zoos and chicken hatcheries offer similar opportunities. The school environment itself should include facilities for keeping pets and breeding wherever it is possible adequately to care for creatures. If facilities are limited it is wise to keep a few animals but offer them as a focal point of learning and exploit this for as long as interest lasts, and then remove them from the school. One often sees animals kept without anything happening which is interesting to the children so that after a while the creatures are not even noticed by them.

Numbers of schools have cats as pets. One two-form entry infant school's cat produced a series of litters which provided talking and learning points. Mostly in groups according to interest there was discussion between children and teacher about the mother cat, for they noticed when she became large. The head-mistress reported:

> I saw some boys playing with her and suggested that they should be gentle as she would soon have her kittens. A small boy added "you mean she is pregnant". The cat has recently been spayed and one of my teachers gave reasons why this was necessary. In the cycle of the school year seeds are sown and tended and tadpoles make an annual appearance so that in many different ways the propagation of life is an idea which we bring in as part of learning.

Another head writes:

> In November last year we had mice and guinea-pigs born in school and the children wrote and talked about "families" and relationships as well as the birth and feeding of the animals.

As part of these topics and probably others too it might, sometimes, also be relevant to talk to children about death. Pets die in

33

school and grandparents die and to come to terms with the first in school could help to come to terms with the second at home. We have tended to hide death from children. We remove the corpse from the classroom quickly and hope the children will soon forget. Yet children are interested in death as well as birth. A gradual understanding of both the beginning and end of life seems now with present knowledge of our own, often inadequate, adjustment to death to deserve serious thought. Certainly a four-year-old boy came to accept the death of a loved grandparent when he came to the conclusion 'Grandpa died to make room for a new baby in the world.'

Children's interest is aroused and maintained when something is happening or developing and there is a marked interest in the birth of young and tremendous pleasure in caring for them (see Fig. 6). Factual learning and emotional and moral growth may well take place simultaneously here, for caring for animals and

Figure 6

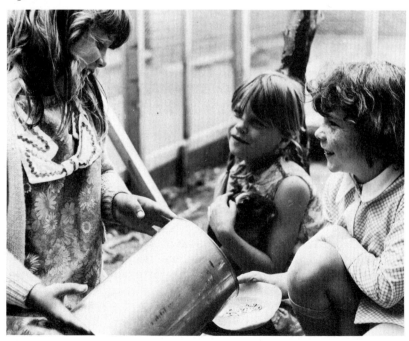

their young affords opportunities for the practice of responsibility and self-control. Here children begin to appreciate that animals in captivity need the best of attention and to keep them and their young is a privilege we should repay.

Yet another headmistress has written:

> Our children take it all for granted. They discuss quite happily the arrival of our various pets (we have gerbils, hamsters, guinea-pigs, rabbits, budgies and fish) and all have offspring fairly frequently! One seven-year-old called me out one day to ask if the frogs were mating and he has asked about the mating of the budgerigars. He also became very involved one day when we were talking (in prayers) about everyone being different and wanted to know how were some twins the same and some quite different and he wanted to know the number of eggs laid by animals and produced by humans.

It is not essential to have animals breeding continuously throughout the school year for children to learn all they wish to know for a period of time. Nor is it desirable to make demands on the same children to be responsible for dependent creatures for too long. In order to keep a soundly balanced curriculum in often crowded primary schools it might be better in some schools to arrange for the young to be born in each spring term, perhaps in two batches. Provided there is real involvement and skilled co-ordinated teaching, the recurring opportunity to experience and learn this annually through the years of the infant and junior schools is likely to be immensely valuable.

Of course where schools have animal houses, covered ways for hutches or covered quadrangles they are better able to incorporate this kind of learning into schools in many different ways.

The Schools Council is currently undertaking a research project into Educational Use of Living Organisms. Booklets on Animal Houses and Small Mammals are in preparation and enquiries should be made to John Wray, Research Fellow, Centre of Science Education, Chelsea College, Bridges Place, London SW6.

Some teachers may feel that one is turning upside down the order in which living things have been traditionally studied in schools. We have tended in the past to start with plants and then move on to the birds and the bees, frogs or rabbits, and finally human beings. Children in some schools never reached the last item before they left school. The order suggested of introducing learning about humans and mammals early comes from our recognition of what is really interesting to children and that is they themselves, their families and creatures who are similar to themselves, particularly small mammals. This will mean that botanical learning involving plant reproduction may more often come later rather than before or parallel with animal and human studies.

Comparing and contrasting newly-acquired knowledge with what is known may also therefore be reversed and will tend to result in comparisons of animals being made with self and other humans rather than learning about human beings by drawing attention to likenesses and differences from the rabbit, rat or frog or African clawed toad, which have been traditionally studied first. This is much more in keeping with the egocentricity of young children and the personal nature of learning in the whole period of the primary and middle school years.

Much efficient, because relevant, teaching in health education is often linked to self-discovery and this comparative egocentricity. Learning could follow on from a cut and bleeding finger with finding out and talking about the blood, the red and white corpuscles, the layers of the skin and the hygienic principles of healing cuts and abrasions.

In running, jumping, hopping and swimming hard the children may become puffed and a simple explanation of respiration could follow and become an introduction capable of further development later. Children may assess their lung capacity and learn something about their lungs, the thorax and the muscles which control inhalation and exhalation.

Development and growth of human beings, of themselves, of babies, toddlers, boys and girls, teenagers, young adults and old people is interesting and draws in children's observation. Good diet for different ages could be included and learning the principles of sound hygiene be started. The series of four books entitled *Growing Up* published by Thomas Nelson have a sound contemporary approach to health education in primary and middle schools and the first book could be introduced at about eight years of age.

Religious education obviously offers opportunities to convey in different ways values related to this area of knowledge to which most of us would subscribe and wish to pass on to children.

Figure 7

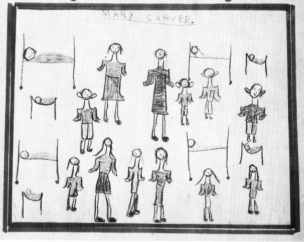

our visit to the
Wokingham Maternity Unit

Figure 8

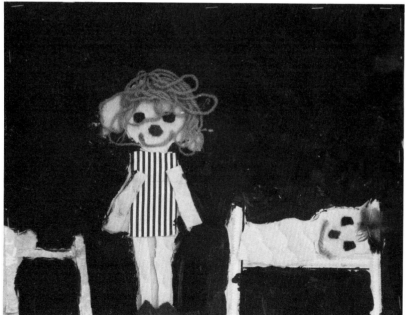

Topics on, for instance, people who care for us could include our mothers and fathers, doctors and nurses, policemen and school crossing warden, etc., and people for whom we can care could include younger brothers and sisters, babies at home and next door, grandparents and other older people (see Figs. 7 and 8).

The learning of moral or religious principles from real life situations lends itself to a study of topics such as these which are relevant to experience and interest provided the teacher takes into account the home circumstances which can influence this learning and skilfully draws on the real life experiences which contribute to the particular learning at any given time.

We have also had occasional assemblies when we have shown the children a family of kittens a few weeks old, a family of young rabbits with their mother and only last week, a supply teacher who is well-known to the children brought her three-month-old baby into assembly and chatted with the children.

Chapter 4

Curriculum for the middle years: eight to ten

It is hardly necessary to point out that education is not divided up into stages by classes, departments or schools but is an all-embracing, continuous process. One of our responsibilities as teachers is to ensure that learning experiences are co-ordinated and that there are no abrupt changes for children in moving from class to class, or from infants to juniors, or from first school to middle school.

The curriculum and vocabulary listed in the previous chapter will certainly be recapitulated and built on with the lower junior age groups and in some schools much of the content may be introduced in the years of seven, eight and nine rather than at five, six and seven. It rests with the head and his staff to plan for the inclusion of this subject when and how it seems best for the particular children in the school.

The difference in the learning between the infant school years and the lower junior years lies in the degree of cognitive development. It can be simply described as being a difference in the degree of understanding of theory and in the complexity of the network of links or relationships which the mind makes between items of theory or knowledge.

Children gradually acquire many different fragments of knowledge and only gradually the ability to perceive relationships and piece the related items together. The mind is rather like a surface for a jigsaw puzzle on which the picture becomes clearer and more comprehensible as more and more pieces are added.

Whereas much of the learning in the infant school period will be incidental and therefore fragmentary—small items of information acquired in many different contexts with some forgotten in one context and remembered through another—the learning of the lower junior school years will be, in a general sense, concerned with an extension of the facts or theory and the gradual fusion of fragmented items of knowledge into a whole. Children are doing this all the time and sometimes coming to wrong conclusions; not because the process of reasoning is faulty, but because their knowledge is inadequate for them to recognise and make accurate links between related aspects of knowledge.

In the area of knowledge with which we are concerned it is not uncommon for children to do this and make such wrong conclusions. One has known of children who knew that a baby grows inside its mother and who heard from a different source that a mother goes to hospital to have a baby. From another source it was learned that one goes to hospital to have an operation and that an operation involves cutting out something bad with a knife. From all this children can come to the conclusion that having a baby must incur a mother being cut open, a kind of caesarian operation. Ideas of birth being through the navel or the anus are also not uncommon.

An important part of learning at about the years seven, eight and nine therefore is to ensure that children have the means to acquire sufficient theory to give the degree of understanding, commensurate with ability, to satisfy curiosity and bring the fragmentary items of knowledge together. Nothing needed for a child's understanding should be omitted. The aim in this subject, at this period of development, can be simply expressed as a gathering together into an orderly sequential body of knowledge the bits and pieces of information learned so far. This body of knowledge will still be comparatively simple but it will be an accurate outline, a firm foundation to which further learning can be added.

The approaches are again, as in the earlier years, as varied as the areas of the curriculum. With skilled teaching this can often be made most meaningful through the approach in which the teacher feels most secure (see Fig. 9). The class teacher with a sound knowledge of biology or health education may extend theory and understanding through topics, studies and projects centred in these areas (see Fig. 10). Another, who is better informed in environmental studies of a more sociological nature, may approach this through a study of the community. Yet another teacher may prefer to incorporate the theory into topics on such subjects as the responsibilities of parents and children to each other, in the context of religious or moral education.

The context itself is not important provided it is of interest to the majority of the children and it can be made a relevant setting for what is important, and that is the sequence of events which make up the story of how we came into the world, how a baby is made and what happened to start a baby growing. This can be a story of most satisfying logic and sense to children of this age. The inclusion of the role of the father is important for it not only accounts for the importance of the father's role in family life, which both boys and girls need to know, but gives the father's part in reproduction so that it is seen as the essential contribution which starts the beginning of a new life and as a part which is vital, apt and logical. It makes sense of the close relationship between parents of which most children will be aware.

The questions the children ask in conversations in homes and schools, where they can speak freely, reveal the sequential nature of their own interest and how the answer to one query leads in time to the next. At about three or four years the interest is in 'Where did I come from?' or 'Where did that baby come from?' Later, perhaps hours, or days, or months, or sometimes years, all quite normal interest is in that part which is framed by the sort of question 'How did the baby get into Mummy's tummy?' and then later again 'How did it get out?'

Cognisance of these factors in children's learning about babies and themselves underlies the BBC radiovision programme 'Where Do Babies Come From?' and the television series 'Beginnings', 'Birth' and 'Full Circle' presented as part of the long-established programme 'Merry-Go-Round' which has been transmitted twice a week for schools on BBC1 for about eight years.

The School Broadcasting Council, composed of educationists of all kinds and representing educational establishments at various

Figure 9

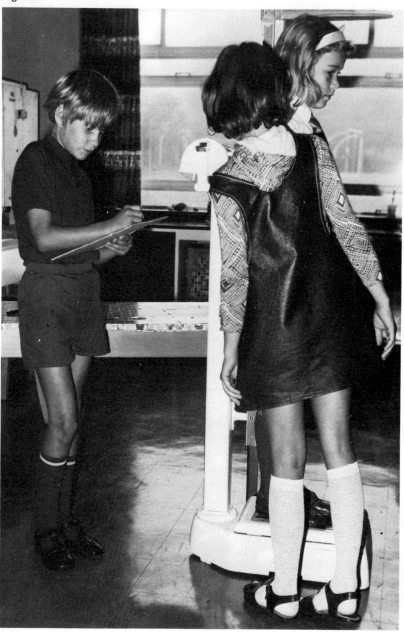

Figure 10

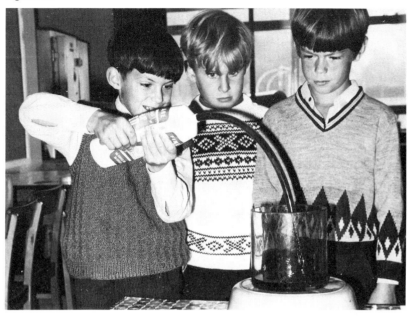

levels, is the body responsible for assessing the needs of the society and its schools in the field of sound radio and television. The Council requested the BBC to examine ways in which these media might help to provide material to assist teachers to extend the curriculum at primary level to include the foundations of sex education.

The radiovision programme 'Where Do Babies Come From?' has seemed to many teachers and parents to be quite the best approach we yet have for bringing together into a wholeness all the fragmentary information the child has acquired by giving him the story of how a baby is born, the sequence of events in logical order. It is an excellent medium for this learning for these reasons. It answers the three questions which children have started to ask from about the age of three. It gives the facts simply, in language which most children easily understand with enough accurate terminology for further learning to take place. It strongly implies the human values we would wish to associate with the theory without explicitly stating moral conditions for family life which could alienate children who do not have both parents, who know themselves to be illegitimate or adopted or know their own circumstances to be irregular. It is a warm and gentle introduction using a fairy story type of illustration with colour and ornamentation around the illustration of each main point to which children can move their attention if they wish. The speed of the commentary and the interaction with the music allows individual internal repetition of each piece of information as the music is played. The material is reasonably priced and can be owned by schools so that it can be shown to children when the time is opportune and as many times as teacher and children wish. It is entirely controlled by the teacher who can stop the programme to give additional information and comment. The teacher's own commentary can be used although one has known of few who felt they could improve on the excellent commentary broadcast in the Nature Series for schools to tape. It can easily be viewed by teachers to familiarise themselves with the content to enable them to make adequate preparation.

The filmstrip 'Where Do Babies Come From?' and the taped commentary can be made relevant to the learning in any school. In those which use the established BBC radio series Nature it quite obviously easily forms a part. It can be equally relevant to any of the approaches suggested above and, if preceded by a simple explanation by the teacher, it can also be a unit of learning in itself. In all these approaches it is important to plan for an adequate length of time for conversation, comment and questions and repetition—immediately after viewing and/or within a few days according to the children's wishes. The outline is simple and some children will want more information than the programme itself offers. Some may reveal their confusions and will want the teacher's reassurance that the story is correct in order to relearn accurately.

This is the actual text accompanying the radiovision programme 'Where Do Babies Come From?' It is given with a small illustration of each frame in the Teachers' Booklet N. 256 obtainable from BBC Publications for Schools. The number refers to the frame and the title describes it briefly. The notes in italics are not part of the commentary but additional information given in the Teachers' Booklet which teachers might find helpful to give to children if they are interested.

1. Man's and woman's heads

Hello. This is a picture of two grown-up people, a man and a woman. There are lots of people in the world, millions in fact, men and women, boys and girls, all different to look at. How did all these people come into the world? That is what we are going to talk about today.

(The population of the world in June 1966 was established by the United Nations to be 3,353 million. By the end of the century the population is expected to be approximately double that, i.e. about six and a half thousand million.)

2. Family group

All the people in the world started off their lives as babies, like the baby you can see here wrapped up warmly in its shawl, and held tightly in its mother's arms. The other person in the picture is the baby's father.

3. Words

But where do babies come from? Turn to the next picture and you'll see.

4. Pregnant woman

From inside their mothers' tummies, that's where babies come from. This lady's going to have a baby. Her tummy is round and big because there's a baby inside. If you had X-ray eyes you could see through her skin to where the baby is, curled up safe and warm.

5. Interior view of pregnant woman

If you had X-ray eyes, this is what you could see inside the lady's tummy. A young baby, just about ready to be born. Inside all women there is a place for babies to grow. It's called a womb. The womb is about half way down from the navel and it's right inside the woman's body, right in the middle. The way out of the womb is through the vagina which ends in an opening between the woman's legs. Where the hair is in the picture.

During the last month of pregnancy the baby usually sinks lower in the pelvis, head downwards, ready for delivery. It is not uncomfortable for the baby to be upside down, because it is floating, not resting on a hard surface. The baby can't fall out of the womb because the cervix, the mouth of the womb, which opens into the vagina, is tightly closed until stretched open by the muscles during labour. Another name for womb is uterus.

6. Girl

Girls have the same sort of insides as grown-up women, but of course they're much smaller. This little girl has a vagina. You can see the outside end of the vagina here. And inside she has a womb, which you can't see because we haven't done an X-ray picture this time.

Girls are born with uterus, ovaries (containing thousands of un-developed egg-cells) and vagina. The vagina is really a passage, protected from the outside by fleshy 'lips' known as labia. Urine does not come out down the vagina. It comes out of the bladder through a tube called the uretha which ends in a separate tiny hole, still within the labia, but higher up and separated from the end of the vagina.

7. Boy

Boys are different, of course. The main difference is that instead of a vagina, they have a penis, and underneath the penis there's a small bag of skin. But the inside of boys is different from girls too. Boys don't have any place for babies to grow.

Boys are born with a penis and a scrotum, which is a small bag containing immature testicles, or testes (the singular of testes is testis). Until puberty it is possible for the testicles to 'migrate' up into the abdomen. After puberty the testicles are permanently descended. In boys, the penis is only used to carry out urine from the bladder.

8. Man

Men look like boys except that they are bigger and have hair growing on various parts of their bodies, like round the penis, and on their chests and faces. The penis doesn't always hang down softly as it does here. It can sometimes become stiff and firm and then instead of hanging down it stands up at an angle. Men can't make a baby grow inside them either. But without men there would be no babies. It takes a man and a woman together to make a baby.

At puberty the penis and testicles develop and the testicles begin to make sperm cells. These are also passed out of the body through the penis. The penis becomes erect because of a flow of blood into the blood vessels in the flesh of the penis.

9. Man and Woman

Grown-up men have a special liquid in their bodies which can come out through their penises. This liquid isn't urine, which also comes out through the penis, but a special, different liquid,

with stuff called sperm in it. Women have eggs inside their bodies
—but not like hens' eggs: tiny, tiny eggs, smaller than a pin's
head. If a father and mother want to have a baby a sperm from the
father has to get to one of these tiny eggs in the mother.

*In a man, sperm cells, commonly known as sperm, are continually
produced in vast numbers by the testicles. They pass out of the body
in a liquid known as semen.*

*In the female about half a million undeveloped egg-cells are present
from birth. Only about two thousand develop, and only one per
month is released, from one or other of the ovaries. This egg-cell has
a very short life. If it is not fertilised within about twenty-four hours
of being released it distintegrates.*

10. Intercourse

The tiny eggs are kept right inside a woman's body, near to the
womb. The only way for a man's sperm to get to an egg is through
the woman's vagina. And the vagina is just the right size for the
penis to fit into, especially when the penis is stiff and firm. This is
how babies are begun, with the father lying very close to the
mother, so that his penis can fit into her vagina.

*During intercourse, about 3ml of semen containing several hundred
million sperm are ejected into the vagina. The sperm move upward
into and through the womb and along the tubes leading to the ovaries.
Conception usually takes place in the tube, when one sperm enters the
wall of a newly released egg. The remaining sperm disintegrate.*

11. Woman

If the sperm from the man has got to an egg in the woman's body
a baby begins to grow. You can't tell straight away that a baby is
growing inside a woman's body, because it takes months to grow
and at first her tummy looks quite flat.

*After conception, the fertilised egg moves into the uterus and begins
to develop by cell division. Signs of pregnancy in the first months
include 1. cessation of menstruation 2. slight enlargement of the cervix
(detected by internal examination) 3. presence in the urine of a
certain hormone which can be injected into frogs causing the frog to
ovulate. Externally, after about twelve weeks the top of the womb
can be felt rising out of the pelvis above the pubic bone.*

12. Pregnant woman

In fact it takes nine months for the baby to grow and be ready
to be born. By the time the nine months are up, the mother's

tummy looks rather like this. Inside the mother there is a real, living baby, almost ready to be born.

13. Words
But how does a baby get out of the womb? How can it get out of its mother's tummy?

14. Birth picture
Well, it comes out quite naturally, usually with a little help from a doctor or nurse. It comes out head first through the vagina, which is very soft and stretchy when a baby is ready to be born. That cord that is joined on to the baby's middle is what the baby got its food through when it was inside its mother. You've got a mark where your cord used to be: that's your navel.

Babies are born about 40 weeks after conception, when the muscles in the walls of the uterus begin to contract. This is called labour. Labour is divided into three stages. During the first stage the contractions cause the cervix to stretch open. During the second stage the baby is born. During the third stage, which is brief, the placenta is expelled. First babies are usually born in hospitals. Later babies are usually born at home. At birth the baby's mouth and throat are cleared of mucus, it takes its first breath and utters its first cry. The umbilical cord is tied in two places and cut in between. This does not hurt the baby or the mother.

15. Baby boy
All babies, right from the very beginning, are either girl babies or boy babies. This one's a boy baby. He has a tiny penis, that's how you can tell. He may grow up to be the father of other babies.

Babies, unlike kittens, can open their eyes as soon as they are born, although they can't see very clearly. They can hear noises. They can smell and taste. They can yawn and sneeze and hiccough. They can suck and burp. Their fingernails and toenails are perfectly developed and they can grip firmly with fingers and toes. They may have hair or not. Their eyes are usually an opaque blue colour.

16. Baby girl
This one's a girl baby. She has a vagina. She may grow up to be a mother.

During the first year of childhood the baby develops the following abilities. About 3 months: holds his head up well, turns his head to look at things and people, smiles. 4 months: begins to make different sounds. 5 months: can pick up small objects. 6 to 7 months: can nearly sit alone. 9 months : perhaps can crawl. 10 months : perhaps can stand up and say one or two words. 12 months : perhaps can walk.

17. Family Group

All the people in the world were made in the way we've told you today, by a man and a woman together. All the people in the world grew first inside their mother's womb, and then were born. And that's where babies come from.

From this will be seen that the following words will be needed for accurate learning in addition to the vocabulary suggested for earlier years.

population	pregnant	pregnancy	
womb	ovum		
scrotum	testes (testis is singular)	semen	sperm
fertilisation	reproduction	generation	
conception	conceive		
foetus	embryo	bladder	

Schools have varied in their timing of the introduction of more formal learning of theory. Some have maintained the incidental approach longer than others but some have introduced theory earlier believing that their children were ready for the whole story in sequential order. In a few schools this has been at the end of their infant school at about the age of seven years.

The majority of schools known to the writer have made, with their parents, what seems to be a safe decision for all children: to introduce a more formal approach towards the end of the first year in the junior school, or the last year of the first school, that is when most children are about eight years of age. This is a safe decision in that we know that the sort of information as in 'Where Do Babies Come From?' and in the books in Appendix A is information which children have wanted to have for a long time, some of it from the age of three or four years, so that they are not being given information they do not want to know. A particular value of the use of filmstrip at this age is that it is not evasive but includes, with a picture of a mother and father embracing, a short account of intercourse in a most appropriate manner for children and in a context where it is presented as the vital part of the story, the act which starts the baby growing. This clear statement of intercourse fits into the theme of the story easily and is being given at a stage in development when the child's emotions are comparatively latent, when he is least likely to be emotionally involved. It is the part of the story of where babies come from which is often omitted because it is the most difficult to explain as it is the most difficult to put into a question. Yet it is important that children should, about this stage, grow up with the father's role clearly explained. An introduction at about eight years or earlier ensures that this is possible. If this information is delayed to the age of nine or ten it is more likely that the introduction will be given with a stronger emotional reaction from the child and the risk that this may inhibit the questioning approach which most eight-year-olds have towards all things which interest them. This may result in individual children getting the facts less clearly and easily than they would do if they had the opportunity to begin to learn them earlier and their curiosity was not hampered by emotional reaction.

Once the door has been opened on this subject as a formal body of knowledge, albeit still but a simple outline, it is important that it remains always open so that it can become part of any other learning which seems relevant. In some schools at present children may need to be shown by their teacher that this subject can continue to be talked about when relevant. This is important for the acquisition of additional theory and for moral education.

An important reason for incorporating this knowledge into primary school work is that it not only provides the foundation for knowledge of the subject itself but allows for an earlier, broader foundation for moral education in relation to it. The formulation of a personal moral code comes for most children at a later stage of development than that reached in primary or middle schools, but just as a body of knowledge is put together from fragmented items of information, so is a moral code derived from influences which have impinged on the individual and his thinking about life from his childhood years. It is a sad reflection on some of us that we have sometimes been most condemnatory of what seemed to be irresponsible sexual behaviour of some young people without asking ourselves what opportunity they had to obtain reliable information and what kind of adult example and influences they experienced from their early years which might have helped them to acquire values which are conducive to personal happiness and a sense of responsibility for others. Morality is not acquired from a few talks and sermons. It again grows little by little from first-hand experience of human relationships in daily life.

The following activities are suggested in the Teachers' Booklet N.175 to supplement and follow on and extend this learning. Many other suggestions will come from children themselves.

weight for boys and girls? Make a graph of the birth weights (see

a. Ask the children to bring along photographs of themselves as babies or collect pictures of babies from advertisements. Make a display. If the children's booklet accompanying this series has been bought by the school, cut up a couple of copies to start this wall display.

b. Ask the children to find out how much they weighed at birth (to the nearest ounce). Is there a difference in the average birth weight for boys and girls? Make a graph of the birth weights (see Fig. 11).

c. Get someone to bring a big doll to school. Have it dressed as a

Figure 11

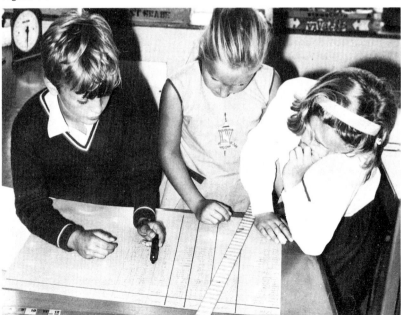

baby. Teach the children how a baby should be held (supporting the head) and how napkins are folded.

d. Make a calendar showing the main events that occur during the first year of a child's life. Find out what foods are eaten by new-born babies, when they begin to eat solid food, when they are able to focus their eyes accurately, when they learn to sit up, when and which teeth come through first, when they first speak.

e. Ask the children to find out what they can about the young of other mammals. What is the gestation period for kittens, puppies, elephants, seals, whales and rabbits? How long is it before each of these stops drinking milk from its mother? What is the average weight of each of these animals at maturity? Is there any connection between weight and gestation period?

f. Keep mice, hamsters, gerbils or rabbits in the classroom or school grounds. Collect frog-spawn and watch it develop. Keep an aquarium and watch water snails or guppies reproduce, or a vivarium in which garden snails and slugs will reproduce. Prepare to rear butterflies at the beginning of the summer term. Incubate a fertilised chicken's egg using a biscuit tin and a 40-watt bulb.

g. See the current Nature teacher's notes for further relevant activities.

'Merry-Go-Round' is a popular and established television programme for schools for the ages of about seven to nine years. It is a stimulus programme in that the school audiences are not treated as passive recipients of information, but encouraged to be active learners in following up all sorts of enquiries, finding out facts, making comparisons, and constructing models to test hypotheses, etc. Large numbers of classes in primary schools take this programme regularly. It is transmitted twice a week. The presenters are familiar figures to the children and the children expect them to be truthful and accurate. They have conveyed information on a variety of interesting subjects, historical topics, mathematics and space technology, etc. as well as on the subject of human beings, and of life.

The three films 'Beginning', 'Birth' and 'Full Circle' form part of a year's 'Merry-Go-Round' programme. They are shown at the close of the academic year when in most circumstances children will have established a relationship with their teacher and be most in control of their learning environment.

This unit of learning could be taken as an introduction to sex education as a central theme from which relevant learning could stem, or be integrated into a class's own scheme of work in various ways. It is believed by the writer, and many teachers, to be most valuable if taken about a year after 'Where Do Babies Come From?' and so build on it to give more detailed information and further extend concept development. The first two programmes cover that part of reproduction which seems to interest children most, that is the growth of the baby *in utero* and birth. Conception comes in the third programme.

In the first programme we see kittens, puppies, chicks and a baby elephant with their mothers. We see two pregnant mothers visit their doctors, we learn that inside the mother is a real live baby with a heart beating faster than an adult's heart. We see a pregnant cat and in a clear outline how her kittens live inside her before they are born. We can learn this again with a mother dog with her unborn puppies and a pregnant woman with her unborn baby. Such information explains simply and in a matter-of-fact manner just what many children want to know to supplement their own observations of pregnancy and in some cases confirm their own ideas or help them to adjust their ideas to reality and accuracy. It is suggested to the children that they find out about the rate of their own heartbeat. All the animals shown are born from inside their mothers except the chick and they are asked to find out how he is born.

The second programme shows a chick pecking his way out of his shell and becoming tired with his efforts. It includes a sequence showing a tabby cat giving birth to her kittens and later the birth of a human baby in diagrammatic form. This is followed by the birth of Stephen whose mother was seen in hospital and walking with Stephen's father and their dog in the first programme. The father's supporting role in the birth of a baby is clearly shown and the beginning of a family portrayed. As in 'Where Do Babies Come From?' this is suggested with great sensitivity, as a fact applicable in Stephen's family and with which children in similar circumstances will identify themselves. But it is not given as an absolute fact applicable to all as an essential condition, a prerequisite for a baby's birth. Much care has been taken not to alienate the child who does not have a normal family but to offer him a picture of, and feeling for, family life, to which he might be attracted and may keep as a desirable ideal as he develops into adolescence.

The third and last programme shows Stephen as a toddler with his baby brother Julian unable to do many of the things he has learned to do. There is sound emphasis on the long time it takes for humans to grow up compared with other mammals in the programme and what a lot humans have to learn. The fact that we are made from part of each parent is made clear with reference to the white and tabby kittens with their tabby mother and white father. The parallel with human beings is made explicit with photographs of faces of mother and father divided into fragments like a jigsaw puzzle and then a photograph of their child showing his own individuality incorporating features of each. Physical differences between baby boys and girls, toddler boys and girls, boys and girls of about nine and ten years of age and adult men and women are shown in sensible situations—bath time and swimming baths for the former and in the still life art studio for the adult figures. Diagrammatic representations of male and female reproductive organs accompany a simple verbal explanation of the way in which the sperm are introduced into the vagina. Microphotography shows the sperm entering the ovum and fertilisation taking place followed by cell division. This is likely to be most easily understood if the child already has a simple idea of intercourse as presented in 'Where Do Babies Come From?' and in books such as *Your Body*, Puffin, *The Wonderful Story of How You Were Born,* Gruenberg, *Time to Grow UP,* Tame, *Right from the Start*, Matthews, so that he is able to make the mental link for himself without the necessity of providing a visual presentation of intercourse which in this more reality-centred material could over-dictate the child's learning in an area where learning is a fusion of feeling and reality. The last sequence shows the family at the seaside with Stephen jumping into a pool of water and Julian in his pram. Most children find this little boy attractive and the scene nearly always evokes pleasure in remembering their own water play in pools or puddles, water troughs and the kitchen sink.

'Where Do Babies Come From?' is the story of how babies are born which takes fifteen minutes to be told. Each 'Merry-Go-Round' programme lasts twenty minutes. It was suggested earlier that 'Where Do Babies Come From?' has seemed the best introduction to the subject we have so far and I am now suggesting that 'Merry-Go-Round's' unit of three films is the best development of this outline that we have. This is because both are child centred and made with the child's idea of the world in mind.

Adults, mostly teachers and parents, who have seen both kinds of presentation with the writer have tended to like one kind of presentation more than another. Views have seemed to be equally divided between the two. This is probably very much to do with whether, as an adult, one finds the style of art in the radiovision attractive or not. The writer's reasons for suggesting that children should be offered both, at different stages in development, are not only that it has seemed that one follows on and enlarges on the content of the first but also because over a long period some children are likely to remember in the terms of one programme and some in terms of the other. Some children may retain a kind of amalgamation of both. Schools which can offer both allow the child a chance to grow intellectually and emotionally on what suits him best. The child is offered both approaches to learning and will retain what is relevant to his own emerging personality.

Although it was suggested that a safe upward age to learn the content of 'Where Do Babies Come From?' was at the end of the first junior year when most children will be about eight years of age or approaching eight and that 'Merry-Go-Round' should be seen about a year later when most children will be about nine, again as in radiovision, some schools have taken this learning earlier and some later. Some schools where young children view 'Merry-Go-Round' regularly have continued with the programme and included the three films for them. The children enjoyed them and talked and discussed the subject fully. It may well be, however, that they will have a greater understanding if it is possible for them to see the same material again when they are about nine. When six-year-olds in a three class family atmosphere school chose to see the programme, with parents' knowledge, and were asked whether they liked it, they answered in the affirmative but said they would like to see it again. This suggests that they themselves knew that they had not fully comprehended the content. Nevertheless the head, teachers and parents were happy that the learning experience had been a constructive one in line with the children's wishes. It had contributed to a desirable situation where learning of this subject is treated incidentally yet purposefully from the beginning and learning can therefore be a gradual thing in line with developmental factors.

'Where Do Babies Come From?' taken with children at about eight years of age is generally accepted as a truthful story. The amount of conversation, writings and drawings and number of questions asked vary, probably according to the follow-up work which stories normally receive. 'Merry-Go-Round' a year later is a denser piece of learning and is so constructed as to encourage children to be active participants. Most schools have a wider range of individual, group and class activities resulting in a large variety of children's work following on from 'Merry-Go-Round' than 'Where Do Babies Come From?'. This is understandable and seems just as it should be. 'Where Do Babies Come From?', though used in many different contexts, is likely to be an introduction of the story-events in order and children will think about it now and again and ideally will follow up points with parents and teachers whenever they wish. After about a year they will be accustomed to the relevance of this subject to all areas of the curriculum. They will be using an accurate vocabulary easily and will be ready for the more complex concepts, or ideas, of the 'Merry-Go-Round' programme and for a greater involvement in the variety of learning experiences it offers.

Teachers will find that children who are accustomed to finding out and communicating information which interests and engages their minds in a variety of ways, will certainly wish to do so here and will model in clay, carve in soap, balsa and salt, make models in papiermâché, and friezes in paint, expanded polystyrene and other media. Writing will be in prose and poetry and often illustrated. Many children will want to follow up certain aspects of the subject in greater detail and good resource books (see Appendix B) will be helpful. Some children like great accuracy, and factors such as the minuteness of the early embryo and its rapid growth fascinate them and they want to record this accurately.

It is fair to say here that schools where children have wished to engage in activities which enable them to re-think and record their learning have had teachers who saw their ways very clearly in this area and always gave children opportunities for initiative and planning as a part of learning on many topics. Some teachers have not had much individual or group work from children as a follow-on to the learning given. This is likely to be because they themselves were unsure of what to suggest and what to provide because they did not have a great deal of experience of working with children in the subject. Some were conscious of the need to respect children's feelings and did not wish to push the facts and re-learning at them. They are surely right to be cautious and to endeavour to preserve a sensitive awareness to children so that there is no intrusion on their deep feelings and privacy. Where this attitude prevails developments are likely to be appropriate, for, after having more experience of working with children in this area, teachers do find ways of sensitively encouraging recapitulation and personal learning and recording by the children without having to put undue pressure on them or intruding upon their personal privacy.

Although not all schools have had group, class or individual projects, topic books or recording in writing or art and craft materials following this learning, all have allowed for discussion incidentally following on from the direct teaching either in class and/or various size groups. They have appreciated that this is of great importance to children and a vital part of learning itself.

It has been clear to us that teachers' confidence and pleasure grow in working with children in this area and they themselves develop with their children an embracing and continuing interest which allows them to explore related fields and recapitulate the factual knowledge and check for accuracy. Teachers will need time to gain this experience but we have found that children's interests bring this quickly.

The following accounts are from a few of the schools who have extended the curriculum to include sex education in various ways. In all these schools the heads had given serious consideration to the importance of personal relationships in education. They also had included sex education in school learning before the availability of the BBC material. The need for such material was felt by them so that as soon as it became available it became incorporated into the school's own scheme of work. All these schools co-operated with parents from the beginning.

The first school is a growing three-class school for five- to eleven-year-olds on the fringe of an ancient university city. The head is the class teacher of the older children whose ages range from nine to eleven. He is an experienced and keen teacher of environmental studies and integrates a great deal of general learning and the acquisition of basic skills into this. He works closely with parents in all areas of the curriculum.

The headmaster writes:

Prior to last year there was no set time for the introduction of sex education other than it was to be included in the curriculum in the final two years. We seemed to enjoy a close relationship within the class and talking freely presented no problems. I felt that the opportunity for sex education would arise quite naturally and as I was the teacher concerned I was sure that no manipulation was needed for it could arise in many ways. This came mostly over frequent observations of selected plots of land where the presence of mating insects caused the talks to begin, usually with small groups. When I passed on to the next groups I would introduce the topic, e.g. 'The last group I visited said that the smaller green nettle beetles are trying to kill the bigger ones'. 'Have you noticed this?' 'Are they fighting?'

On the return to class I would talk to them about the life and life cycle of the creatures we had discovered. At this time I stated that during the days to follow we would talk about animals, including man, and asked if anyone could find any information, would they please collect it together with books on the subject from the school library and home. I was surprised by the number of children that had books on the subject at home.

I took the approach—your parents I am sure *will* have told you, but to ensure that it has been fully understood we will go through it once more.

Before the second talk I would remind the class about pictures of Victorians bathing, Victorian children dressed for a day by the sea which was part of a topic we had studied. We would then discuss how lucky we are with our freedom to dress suitably, we'd also talk about changing attitudes, how strange (laughable) we should find their manners and standards of rigid behaviour. Victorians and much more recent generations were unable to talk about many subjects— e.g. the very thing we had talked about only that week would have been impossible—were not these strange attitudes to have?

Tolerance, understanding and correct behaviour towards others of different creeds, colour, belief, modes of dress, I believe has to be one of the most important attitudes to be learned today—this I stress here and in school continuously. The children accept that the nakedness of a child in Africa is only embarrassing to us because we are unused to nakedness and no one has ever seemed too embarrassed to talk freely during the talks on personal relationships.

At this time other teachers were informally asked to talk as freely as they felt able to when answering the questions that would arise from keeping pets and studying animals.

We received no criticism and no whisper of objection.

Last year when it became available I decided to use the 'Merry-Go-Round' Series with all the children in the eight to eleven age group, and was therefore for the first time given a fixed date when preparation had to be complete. We were also introducing a new relationship or a third party into our discussion in the person of Richard Carpenter, the presenter.

The series you may recall received some publicity—local newspapers carried such column headings as, 'Parents to decide says Headmaster'. I would, I think, have shown the series as part of our established programme of work for we were not showing the children how to forge money or pick pockets—but with all the local and national publicity I felt obliged to consult with parents and explain our approach. The parents of one child out of over sixty children asked for the child to be withdrawn from the lessons.

Our introduction began when we borrowed an incubator from our local College of Education. A series of experiments were carried out and eggs from various sources were used. The most successful eggs were those purchased from a farm which sold guaranteed fertile eggs. Why were they fertile?

The work was most exciting and rewarding. A great deal of work arose from this, e.g. temperature analysis, increase in weight graphs, increase in size, weight of food used, cost of food—return in value, stages of development, diaries of growth, care of animals, etc.

Our children were well adjusted but the poor chicks, which had been kept separately for various reasons, were less clear about parenthood and would have nothing to do with their own kind; they followed their proud keepers in a hilarious and devoted manner around the school field and yard.

One needs patience and strong nerves when one has piping chicks in the classroom and finally a hard heart when one parts with them after ten or twelve weeks.

When the number of chicks increased, they were taken

home at weekends by children. One afternoon I received an excited telephone call from a child—'Please come over, Mr ———,' but she would not give any further explanation. I travelled a total of twenty miles, the six-week-old chick was gently lifted up and there nestled in the sawdust was one of the smallest pullet's eggs I have ever seen. 'Isn't it wonderful, Mr ———?' said Mum. It was most difficult to remind the parent that it was April the First and I had caught sight of an old gardener with wicked eyes and a schoolboy sense of humour watching from the other side of the fence.

Observations of the plots of land were still carried out but on reflection I think the preparatory talks, the keeping of animals, were more helpful to our work than the previous method of letting the topic arise.

As the time of the TV 'Merry-Go-Round' programme approached in June I had some doubts. I wondered if we would obtain the same air of frankness or whether the introduction of this other outside party would break down communications and cause discomfort. Fortunately, the programme fitted in perfectly, my fears were unfounded, and the programme's success was unquestionable.

If the climate within the class is right, sex education is natural. I am not so certain that every classroom is always the right place. There is also the moral side which must be discussed and this needs care when there is likely to be present the child born to an unmarried mother. There is also the relationship between parents and love which needs to be included.

I think sex education has its place in the primary school curriculum, but the freedom for the child to talk to parents too is essential.

This year we are borrowing an observation beehive from the College of Education—the social set-up should give rise to some interesting work.

Another school is a new one-form entry school for five- to eleven-year-olds serving an urban area of recent housing development with good rail links to London and a number of commuters among parents. Much of the school work is organised for co-operative teaching of different kinds. The headmaster of this school writes:

The parents were consulted so that we could judge their willingness to support us in arranging for their children to take part in discussion and instruction on human reproduction and life and their views of how and when this should be done. I felt that if the subject was to be given it would best be done with the co-operation and goodwill of the parents and that careful consideration should be paid to their views. I asked all parents who could if they would view the programme 'Merry-Go-Round' on television and I also purchased the filmstrips 'Growing Up' and 'Where Do Babies Come from?'. I showed the filmstrips to the largest single gathering of parents we have ever had and then we split up into discussion groups. The result of this was that they came down very heavily in favour of including sex education but that it should be carefully introduced in smallish groups and perhaps in detail in the third or fourth year, nine to eleven years. First-year children saw the 'Merry-Go-Round' films.

We had already a syllabus of science in the third and fourth year team that included some Human Biology (Respiration, Circulation, Food, Growth, and so on) and it was possible to include sex education into this. The science is taken in the learning unit by the deputy head who extracts groups of about twelve children at a time. They perform tasks, experiments, watch films and filmstrips, e.g. 'Working Water', Dowling Films Production from Sound Services, etc., in the normal course of events, so the introduction at the suitable point of the two radiovision filmstrips passes without special notice. We use them because they fit well with the approach to science that we use and are readily available. Full discussion and comment is encouraged and a matter-of-fact attitude of concern has been adopted in answering questions. The children are never in larger groups than about a dozen when the topic of sex is introduced or the filmstrips shown and we have been most careful to look out for any distress. To date no children have been reported to be suffering from nightmares or other worry symptoms and we have not seen any worry in school. We try to obviate this by careful introduction and lead up anyhow, and as far as we know there has been no 'sniggering in the corner'. We have had no complaints from parents, a number of thanks and some compliments.

The sociological aspects of procreation within the family unit achieve the main emphasis, for example, the nurture that we receive, our body being fed, clothed and protected, growing up and leaving home, ourselves marrying and having babies, death and disposal, and then a switch back to where we came from, and what happens when and as we grow up. The children take this in their stride and they really do approach it in the same manner as though it was 'William the Conqueror' or 'Brunel's Bridges'. Here are two examples of comments during conversation that give some indication of their thinking:

1) During discussion on ovum and spermatozoa.
    Boy Isn't it amazing how tiny the egg is that babies come from?
    Girl Yes. Have you seen that tiny box that Jenny's Dad brought home from Hong Kong?
2) *Girl* Sir, I read in the paper that girls of fifteen who were not married were having babies.
    Boy They don't have to be married to have babies.
    Girl Yes, I know, but it means that the babies are born without Dads. How terrible not to have a Dad.
    General murmurs of assent.

Discussion arises spontaneously from the children and can also be guided by, for example, stopping the tape and the strip at a particular frame during the showing of the filmstrips. The choice of frame is important. The one depicting the birth of a baby occasions a great deal of enquiry, e.g. the length of the cord, whether a baby is always born head first, and so on. I should hesitate to stop at the frame depicting the embrace during intercourse for fear that some difficult questions were asked. This is personal, of course, and merely shows my own inadequacy at present. It may not cause any problems to others particularly with experience of this topic.

The questions that parents ask spring mainly from the fear that children will learn the physical facts of sex without due consideration given to emotional aspects. They fear that extra knowledge will lead to lax behaviour and that information will be given without value judgments. 'Are you going to mention marriage?' 'Are you going to stress the importance of love and security?' were asked and we were able to assure them on these points.

At the beginning teachers' questions to me came from uncertainty of limits and knowledge. 'How much detail must I give?' They need to know that explanations of detail are unnecessary and a simple answer is all that is required. Young teachers asked 'How do you talk about love and sex if you have not experienced it yourself?' 'How much value is there in doing just the biology part?' Young teachers realise that children too will have no opportunity of love and sex but will want to have the sort of information that the young teacher needed too at their age. Many young teachers can remember their own needs.

I see the task of the head and his staff as that of imparting essential knowledge, and instilling reasonable attitudes towards sex.

Our main source material are books and filmstrips. The books that we have are:

Peter and Pamela Grow Up	H. W. Tame
Time to Grow Up	H. W. Tame
Your Body and You	Junior True Book
Health	Junior True Book
How the Baby Came	D. Allen and M. Neurath
How John Grew an Inch	D. Allen and M. Neurath
Keeping Well	M. Neurath
Health and Hygiene	British Red Cross Society

In this school the children at the end of their first year in junior departments saw 'Merry-Go-Round' which forms the introduction to the more detailed work outlined above. The deputy head concerned with the detailed work writes:

I was only indirectly aware of what happened to the 'Merry-Go-Round' viewers: passing through the classroom when the programme was on I noted rapt faces and keen attention. A little diplomatic eavesdropping in the break gave no indication of 'smutty' or 'silly' reminiscences. I heard only a fierce debate as to whether the baby was born head first or feet first, a debate which changed tack in the best tradition of primary polemic progressing through the birth of puppies, on to the manner in which a dog enters and leaves a kennel — does he come out backwards? Then: 'My dad was reversing out the other morning . . .' the conversation bubbled and shifted and heaved about like yeast.

Opponents of sex education must, I think, forget the youngster's lively and divergent mind, his transience, his fleeting interest—for the moment—in the matter of the moment. Among a pile of newspapers someone in my class found a weekend supplement with a colourful account of a caesarian birth. He brought it to me, and in tow were a couple of interested companions.

As we discussed the illustrations a group of half-a-dozen boys and girls gathered round me. The general view was that it was 'great'. Someone expressed surprise that a baby should be so big at birth; he was immediately informed by a class-mate that they started 'very, very small'. 'How small, Sir?' 'Well,' I said, 'I believe the mother's egg is about the size of that full stop'. 'Did you see,' they asked me, 'that tiny dictionary that Jane had, only the size of a matchbox, or less?' That too, if misleadingly, was judged to be 'great', and the group split up, some to seek out the legendary Jane, others to admire the Lord's Prayer engraved on the pendant of Anne's necklace. Anne was one of the trio who, scarcely five minutes before, had brought me the colour supplement. Was this a trivial, trite and useless encounter with birth? Not at all; the group all recalled it, later, during a conversation following one of the BBC radiovision programmes. And it was their reaction to just that sort of encounter that helped me to decide to present to my nine- to eleven-year-olds these two programmes. Parents when consulted were agreeable to the idea and often grateful.

The first, 'Where Do Babies Come From?', consists of a filmstrip of 16 pictures and a taped commentary which runs for a quarter of an hour.

The presentation begins with a reference to a family group and goes on to show, as if with X-ray eyes as the speaker puts it, the unborn baby. A far cry from these very inelegant, if factual, technical illustrations of the womb, this picture, like the other frames in the filmstrips, is gently drawn and delicately coloured. There is just a hint of the whimsical about many of the pictures, but this is no device for withholding information: rather a gracious attempt to portray what most educators know to be a subject of simple fascination and wonder for most children.

The commentary is in the same gentle, unemotional vein, and the speaker's voice is ideal, unhurried, matter-of-fact and not in the least condescending or patronising. The words of the subject—penis, vagina, sperm and so on—are used; why not? Children will always find some word, somehow, for the anatomy and the act, and how much easier it will be, as they grow up, to be able to speak confidently and unambiguously to a parent, a friend, the doctor; to be able to read and to understand.

Whatever views there may be on informing youngsters of the process of getting and having a baby, there can be no logical argument against the presentation of the other programme, 'Growing Up'. With the same clear but not 'clinical' style of illustration this discusses in the same gently helpful manner the bodily changes that a boy or girl will experience as part of growing up. I used both productions with mixed groups, keeping the numbers to about a dozen for ease of discussion.

Both boys and girls were obviously grateful for the simple facts of menstruation, and became absorbed in studying the development of the unborn baby. Such discussion and inquiry would of course have gone on somewhere, and probably already had, however furtive and ill-informed the occasion. As their teacher I was happy to be able to help to put the record straight and I felt rather privileged to be included in the discussions of these young people.

Sex 'education' of some sort is inevitable, and illegitimate babies are not the invention of the twentieth century. Nothing but good can come of the informed use of programmes of education such as primary schools now have available.

In another one-form entry school for five- to eleven-year-olds the first and second year juniors still work in the old school in the centre of the village. The rest of the school occupies a new school on the outskirts of the village in the midst of new, mostly local authority, housing. The infant department under an older deputy head is organised in three classes with some use of a shared activity area. The junior school is organised for co-operative teaching; the first and second years in one unit for learning and the third and fourth years in another. The head himself teaches more than half the week. He is interested in programmed learning and other ways of encouraging independent learning although this is only an addition to teacher guided work and one of a variety of teaching methods used. The headmaster writes:

1. **Outline of our Approach**

a) Infants
Little is deliberately introduced except through the rearing and observation of small mammals. We are reduced to gerbils only, at present, but I do regard these as being a most useful subject as they exhibit such strong 'family' awareness. Questions are freely answered as they arise and discussions ensue from time to time on such occasions as the arrival of a new baby in a family, or if kittens, etc. are born.

b) Lower School Team (first and second year juniors)
(i) Continued observation of mammals. This will be more directed during this coming summer term.
(ii) Investigation and discussion of various forms of reproduction, especially reptilian (good old frog-spawn!).
(iii) Beginnings of biological science with special reference to human biology. This will be part of an overall theme on man. Motivation point—thermatic core, 'Moving' —————— developed 'Man moving' —————— Muscles —————— Skeleton.
(Aids . . . Model–'Visible Man' manufactured by Renivall (U.S.) Ltd. obtainable from toy and model shops and a real skeleton (borrowed from secondary school).

Approach is by:
Group discussions.
'Outline' cards. (Type of assignment card.)
Simple linear programming.
(Teachers are advised to look for means of introducing the duality of biological systems.)
'Merry-Go-Round' programmes.

Opportunities to extend (iii), as above, are looked for, but are not deliberately engineered. Any genuine indications of interest would, however, be followed up in a structured way using:

a) Literature. *Your Body* Ladybird Publication
Jill Kenner's *Where Do Babies Come From?* N.M.G.C.
This is taped as a talking book and can be used by individual children or with small groups using a junction box.
Programmed Sex Information, Books 1 and 2 Kind and Leedham, published by Longman

b) Other material. Work cards, 'How Life Begins', Galt.
Radiovision Strip and Tape 1. 'Where Do Babies Come From?' 'Let's talk about ourselves' Strip 1 and Tape. (Camera Talk series). Model 'Visible Woman' manufactured by Renivall (U.S.) Ltd. and obtainable from most toy and model shops.

The books above, with some others, are always available in the library at all times.

c) Upper School Team (third and fourth year juniors)
i) Continued observation of small mammals, with frequent informal questioning on behaviour. The aim is to establish common factors of mammalian behaviour.
ii) The children progress through linear programmes (taped for aural support), linking these to the current thermatic core if it is appropriate to interest. If such a link is not apparent to the children, the programmes are offered as part of a systematic stimulus for learning as a subject itself. We have planned a sequence of programmes which 'blankets' the reproductive system between other biological systems. The sequence is frequently broken with individual children if interest diverts them on to other studies. Children are assigned one programme per fortnight, and seem to enjoy and benefit from the activity, probably because of the high rate of 'success'. They can consult and talk with the teacher at all times. The planned programme relevant to this area of learning is:
Programme S3. Skeletal system
        S4. Food

S5. Teeth } Logical continuation
S6. Digestion } of S4.
S7. Composition of blood } 'Blanketing'
S8. Circulation of blood } programmes
S2. Cells
S9A. Asexuality and Sexuality
S9B. Anatomy of Reproduction
  Radiovision I (strip and tape)
    'Where Do Babies Come From?'
  Camera Talks
    'Let's talk about ourselves' I (strip and tape)
S9C. Physiology of Reproduction
  Radiovision II (strip and tape) 'Growing Up' 'Let's talk about ourselves' II (strip and tape) Camera Talks
S10. Muscular system }
S11. Respiration } Further
S12. Excretion } 'Blanketing'
S13. Nervous system } programmes
S14. Senses }
S9D. Plant Reproduction also still in preparation (To follow S9C.)
  Simpler versions of S9A, S9B, S9C are to be prepared for younger juniors and less able children, although the existing versions have been used with complete success by children of VRQ's between 90 and 95. I intend these programmes to incorporate a wider use of illustration, but am awaiting a new spirit duplicator.

'Merry-Go-Round' television
iii) Support materials
As for the lower school, also we now use Kind and Leedham's Book 3. Children are directed to the 'Visible Woman' model to ensure that anatomical facts are correctly understood.

Programmes S3 and S4 have, this school year, been withdrawn to make time for the 'Farming' theme. This theme has helped to reinforce the concept of 'mammalianism' and has brought an investigation of poultry reproduction. I think it is likely to arouse interest on heredity but we shall see.

2. Children's Work

a) In connection with the current (1971) farming theme, one group of children, in their weekly report to the rest of the team, has, spontaneously, drawn comparisons between pollination and animal fertilisation.

b) Some Creative English emerged last year. The two samples enclosed resulted from a straightforward weekly assignment including the set subject 'Life Awakens'.

c) A mathematics problem evolving from the phenomenon of cell division has emerged. Originally offered as part of an 'enrichment' display to stimulate interest in the cell it has proved a very useful and successful means of dealing with powers and indices.

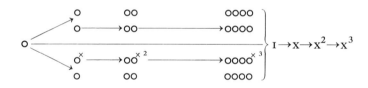

$$1 \rightarrow x \rightarrow x^2 \rightarrow x^3$$

d) As our work is mainly programmed and yet informal and our aim to integrate sex education into any relevant part, no particular emphasis is laid upon this aspect of human behaviour, we get little feedback, apart from instances as in (a) above. Questions are asked incidentally at all sorts of times and we have not had a detailed discussion time arise when a large group discussed the subject together. Last year I engineered discussion with fourth year children, but felt that this was not quite the right approach for our kind of organisation.

e) Several children have, during this school year, taken home programmes, to work and discuss with their parents. So far I have not ascertained reactions from parents, but the children seem happy with this procedure.

Creative English based on set subjects from an assignment entitled 'Life Awakens!' (May 1970):

BIRTH

A new life
Bursts upon the world
A new voice
Cries a message
To the world
A child is born, a young mother is made,
And she has made
A new life
In the world
From the love of two people
Man and Woman
A life created
Now urging forth
From the dark, warm womb
Into a cold day.

EGG

Are you a chick unborn?
Or just another breakfast?
Is there, inside your fragile shell
A wee red speck which tells
That you are alive, waiting.
Waiting to divide, grow, hatch
Into a yellow, furry, pretty thing?
A wee red speck which tells us
You were fathered
By the proud cock, farmyard's king,
A fertilised, living cell, alive,
Waiting to divide, grow, hatch.

The above indicates the way our work started and developed over the last few years.

Now I think there is one point I would like to make—with the early maturing of several top junior girls, and their definite interest in the subject becoming personalised, I have come to the conclusion that my own particular course, which is biologically and scientifically biased, and, to some extent, clinical, should be timed to reach completion before the end of the third junior year and certainly no later than the end of the first term of the fourth year. My theory, and I may be wrong on this, is that once reproductive processes are understood, they can be 'tucked away' into the subconscious. Thus, factually equipped, the children will approach the phenomena of puberty, and such attendant factors as the appreciation of sexual motivation and morality with attendant strong mental processes, more objectively, once the physical processes are accepted as natural functions at an earlier stage of maturation. In other words my whole aim is to ensure children understand essential facts before becoming sexually conscious.

Three examples of this school's programme for individual learning which are particularly relevant are S9A, The Reproductive System, S9B, Anatomy of Reproduction, and S9C, Physiology of Reproduction are given in Appendix E.

The following account is of some work in a two-form entry junior school in a borough near enough to London to have many commuters living in the school's catchment area. The account is given by the deputy head as the head herself is no longer with the authority. The deputy too is now headmaster of a primary school within the same authority. He writes:

The decision to introduce sex education into the curriculum was only taken after a long period of consultation and dialogue between the head, staff and parents. Initial staff response was wary, 'a good idea in principle so long as I'm not expected to do it' seemed the most usual opening response. However, after several periods of discussion, all staff (11 full time plus two part time), except one, agreed to the principle and to participate themselves if asked to do so.

The next stage was to hold meetings for parents. Two of these were held. At the first the radiovision strips on 'Where Do Babies Come From?' and 'Growing Up' were shown and the head and LEA adviser spoke to parents. At the second meeting, the film of the BBC Merry-Go-Round programmes 'Beginning' and 'Birth' were shown. Parents were unanimously in favour of the films but several had definite reservations about the radiovision filmstrips. Only one parent objected to sex education in school, but even she did not withdraw her child from the lessons.

Preparation for the programmes was left to the individual class teachers involved, as was the follow-up work. The reasons here were:–

1. They were the people in closest contact with their particular groups of children and with whom the children would converse most freely.
2. To have changed the 'routine' by having a specialist teacher or head teacher to take these lessons would have defeated the object of keeping the lessons a normal part of the school day and have made them 'special' or 'unusual'.
3. The head felt it impossible to lay down an approach as each teacher approaches all subjects in a different way and would only feel comfortable and build the right atmosphere if using their own approach.

In my own case the programmes were integrated into a study of plant, insect, bird and animal life which evolved from our current river study based on Ray Mill Island. As we discussed the growth and life of plants, so birds, animals and eventually humans were drawn in. The programmes were watched and we held a discussion afterwards. Follow-up work included growth graphs (height/weight of brothers/ sisters of varying ages, of selves and of parents), guessing who's who from baby photographs, comparison of growth rates of birds, animals, humans, dependence of human babies on parents and parental care of children, of birds and animals. Groups also branched out into work on food and diet and variety of homes throughout the world.

I myself found no embarrassment amongst the children. They were interested in the programmes and on the whole were satisfied with the facts given in them. Their comments and questions embraced personal aspects, e.g.

'I was a seven month baby!'
'What does that mean?'
'It means he was premature.'
(Discussion with eleven-year-olds)
'Why do men doctors examine women?' (Martin)

indignant cries from the rest of the class
'Because most doctors are men!'
'My Auntie's baby died, it was choked by the cord'
(Martin again)
'When a baby is born the wrong way round, it's called a breech birth, isn't it?' (Debra)

The most useful book I came across was *Where Do Babies Come From?* by Jill Kenner, published by the National Marriage Guidance Council. Other books were available on the shelves and some were taken home. Some parents reported back to us that this presented them with an excellent and natural opportunity for a discussion with their child.

Of course, it really goes without saying that the success of any attempt at introducing sex education depends on the complex personal relationships within a school. There must be trust and understanding between head and staff, staff and parents and, most important, between the individual teacher and the children with whom he/she is concerned. The teacher must be not only willing but thoroughly prepared to discuss everything with the children. There must be no evasion as this would foster wrong attitudes and ignorance which we hope to dispel.

I'm sorry that I have no actual children's work to send to you but, in moving, I got rid of all that I had saved as one can so easily just carry on accumulating piles of work in the hope that they may, one day, prove useful. We prepared as thoroughly as we were able and then dealt with each situation as it arose. From the reactions of staff, parents and pupils I would say that in our particular situation and with the boys and girls we had, our way of meeting the challenge of providing sex education was successful.

The first three schools whose work is described had established approaches and schemes of work of which sex education was part and they incorporated BBC material into them. The fourth school began to give more attention to sex education than before when the BBC material became available although relevant contexts for it were already established in schemes of work.

The following account is from a two-form entry junior school with a headmistress of many years' experience. She had given serious consideration to sex education and to personal relationships and had read widely on the subject. She saw her way to extend her curriculum when the BBC material became available. The following account shows how she did this and how she and her staff created situations where such learning was appropriate and where children could ask all the questions they wished with ease. She writes:

> I am sorry I have been rather a long time in sending my observations on our personal relationships programme and in particular the sex education films, but I have waited to see the reaction of parents of first-year children who of course did not see the films last year and others where the children have been admitted to second, third and fourth year classes during the year. I can only say that I am delighted with the over-all picture of things and put my findings in this brief report. Unfortunately I was away for a whole month this year while the television programme 'Merry-Go-Round' was taking place, otherwise more might have been done in following up children's interests.
>
> The procedure adopted was as follows:
>
> 1. A letter was sent to all parents of both the junior and infant school inviting them to a meeting on May 11th at which the LEA adviser was the speaker and the programmes were seen. There was a packed hall and many interesting questions were asked by parents.
>
> 2. Immediately after the meeting, on the same evening, many parents approached me and everyone who did so was very impressed with the films. Some favoured the 'Merry-Go-Round' television films, whilst others preferred the radiovision programme, 'Where Do Babies Come From?' and 'Growing Up'.
>
> 3. A few days later this letter was sent to parents.
>
> Dear Parents,
>
> ### Personal Relationships
>
> Following the meeting on Monday evening, I am now wishing to hear the opinions of parents on this subject.

I was very pleased indeed to see such a large number of parents and only wish that all of you could have been there. I feel Mrs ——— talked very well indeed on this matter.

The 'Merry-Go-Round' films are to be shown towards the end of this term and probably the radiovision filmstrips as well.

Would you kindly answer the following questions and return the letter to school? A form *must* be returned for each child.

1. Did you come to the meeting on May 11th? Yes or No.

2. Have you any objection to your child seeing the films? Yes or No.

Remarks : ....

Name of Child
Parent's signature ....

Yours sincerely,

Head Teacher.

P.S. If any parents would like to discuss the matter further with me before signing the form, I would be very happy to see them, particularly if they have not seen the films.

The replies showed this result, that 303 out of 306 children saw the 'Merry-Go-Round' film. I was able to persuade a few other 'hesitants' who had previously said no.

4. The Headmistress then gave a preparatory talk to each class in turn and many interesting questions were asked by the children. There were no signs of embarrassment or sniggering. I was very happy with the children's reaction.

5. The television films were duly seen by the children in 'Merry-Go-Round'—first and second years on one day and third and fourth years on the other day. Sensible questions were asked and answered by those teachers whom I felt sufficiently experienced to be in charge.

There was a follow up in the classroom, generally of a simple nature, particularly information brought from home about weight at birth—where born, etc. I felt that to continue the theme for a prolonged period was not a good idea.

6.   This year this letter has been sent to all parents of first-year children who, of course, were in the Infant Department last year.

Dear Parents,

Personal Relationships

Towards the end of this term you may be aware that on one of the television programmes ('Merry-Go-Round') there will be a series of three lessons on Sex Education (a repeat of last year's *programme*).

Last year I sent out invitations to parents of this school and the infant school to attend a meeting addressed by ————, one of the County's Primary School Advisers. The result of this meeting was that only *three* parents withdrew their children from the lessons, and in the first year *no* child was withdrawn.

I may add that I have been very happy indeed with the reaction of the children. It exceeded all that I could possibly have wished for. Parents have been asked for their reaction and any which I have received have been very favourable. Some parents who were at first a little apprehensive were completely happy with the results.

May I assure you that before the films are shown the children will be adequately prepared so that they are received in the right spirit.

After a great deal of thought I have decided that the film is best shown to first-year children who take it in their stride and are impressed by the wonder of all they see and hear. I favour this age *rather* than the second year where emotionally it *could* mean more to some children.

I hope that once again as last year every parent of this age group will be happy to let the child see the film. There is the obvious situation that if one or two remain outside their curiosity may lead them to find out from other children what the film was about.

Will you kindly sign the form below? I shall be very

pleased to discuss this matter with any parent who wishes to know more. Will you kindly signify in the form if you wish this?

Yours   sincerely,

Headmistress

I wish   .. .. to see the film
I do not wish   .. .. to see the film

Signed:

In addition a letter was sent to all children in second, third and fourth years who were not on the roll of the school when the 'Merry-Go-Round' films were seen. The result of these letters is that every child in the first year is to see the film without question and for the rest of the school all children present who have returned forms have been allowed to see them.

7.   A full range of books is in the school library.

The headmistress of this school, like the majority of heads, has gone to great trouble to help parents to understand the reasons for the school's policy as this letter to a parent of a child in her school shows.

Dear
    I am now in a better position to answer your letter of 17th instant.
    I am pleased that both you and your wife attended the meeting on the 11th as you are better able to express your thoughts on this very important matter.
    Having now perused 306 forms received from parents I have a fairly clear picture of parents' views and reactions to the films. The overwhelming majority are in favour—only five parents to date are unwilling for their children to see them. (I anticipate that this number will be reduced when I have had the opportunity of speaking to the parents concerned.) Whilst six other parents were a little apprehensive about sex education in primary schools many parents expressed the view that the films were excellent and tastefully

presented. They were very happy that schools were helping them in this particular field.

Regarding your point about where responsibility lies for this instruction I suppose most people would agree that it is in the home, but unfortunately statistics show that a high percentage of children do not receive this at all, while many children make their discoveries from very unsatisfactory sources. However, I feel that schools also can play their part.

My decision to show the films has been taken only after hearing parents' views spoken to me personally and on seeing the result of the letter sent out and of course my own convictions on this matter. Comparing the two programmes, 'Merry-Go-Round' and Radiovision, many parents preferred the latter, and would have liked it shown first, though this will not be the case; others however hold your view.

Regarding further meetings I do not feel this to be necessary. Mrs. ——— herself says that the programme should be introduced quite naturally and without too much fuss.

I myself am giving a preliminary talk to each age group in turn. My purpose in doing this is to ensure as far as possible that the children approach this whole subject without embarrassment and in the right spirit. There is far too much unhealthy talk and sniggering, kept well underground, which many of us do not seem to realise. I am anxious to stop this and I feel I shall be better able to assess the attitude of children and their reactions if we are talking openly. Any unpleasantness will be brought to the surface and more easily detected.

The films are to be shown on TV on Mondays, June 1st, 8th and 15th for 7–9 age group and Thursdays, June 4th, 11th and 18th for 9–11 group.

Perhaps you will let me know how you feel about *———seeing the films after reading this letter.

Yours sincerely,

Head Teacher.

8. Radiovision filmstrips and tapes are to be shown this term to the children in the fourth year.

The Head's general remarks. I am entirely happy with the reaction of children in the school. They have just taken it all in their stride. In my mind there is no doubt that this is the stage at which to introduce the subject. I feel that Secondary Schools should go on from here and in particular at about the age of 13 plus. The reaction of parents has, I think, more than proved that they are in full agreement with all that has taken place.

P.S. Sorry I cannot supply material and work of children as this has not been kept.

Chapter 5

Curriculum in the upper junior/ middle school: ten to twelve

As suggested on page 39 learning is a continuing process. Some children will learn much of the curriculum outlined in the previous chapter at a later stage of around ten to twelve years while others will learn it earlier. Here, as with all learning, we shall need to provide for the child to recapitulate, check, test and relearn in his own good time by having the resources and media for this available and by maintaining an atmosphere where he is free to ask directly or otherwise show his need.

An important part of the theory of the story of human life, 'the story of me', has hardly been touched on as so far outlined in this curriculum. This is because the content has tended to concentrate on the information about babies which seems to interest primary school children most. Towards the ages of ten to eleven years, however, this centre of interest slightly changes. We move gradually away from babies and towards an anticipation of future roles. It then becomes desirable gradually to modify the approach from a personal recapitulatory one to one which assists and meets the interests of children who are starting to project forward in thinking and feeling into adolescence. Growing awareness at this time creates a need for factual information about growth and the physical and emotional changes of adolescence as part of normal development of all human beings. This knowledge is a preparation for the changes which lie ahead so that boys and girls are able to understand the changes in themselves as they discern them physically and emotionally in themselves and others.

We know from the research of Professor J. M. Tanner and others that physical maturity in both boys and girls is being reached earlier now than ever before and that with continual improvement in diet and general health this is likely to be maintained. More girls now begin to menstruate while still in primary school. Unfortunately it is not unusual for this to begin in school hours and for it to come as a great shock to the girl. In these circumstances a teacher or head has to try to ameliorate this.

Because of past attitudes we, ourselves, have grown up accustomed in varying degrees to regard the years of adolescence as being years of difficulty and strain, not only for the emerging adults themselves, but also for their parents and teachers and others concerned with their welfare. It may well be that, by comparison with the years of latency, this is so, but knowledge of the findings of anthropologists like Margaret Mead and Ruth Benedict show us that some other societies have managed to contain this period of life within the full time span and make the transition from childhood to adulthood with less difficulty than is achieved by many young people in our society. Reasons for this situation are of course most complex. Nevertheless part of our difficulties may lie in the traditional attitude of many homes and schools which results in failure to acknowledge the changes of these years with little attempt to talk sympathetically with the young about them. It may well be that it is our practice of ignoring the changes of these stages of development which have helped to create a barrier between adolescents and adults. This is understandable, for many of us have lacked the vocabulary to talk easily about human emotions and behaviour with our children even in the early years, so that by adolescence there has been a period of long silence which becomes too difficult to break.

We now know, without doubt, that anxiety builds up in these years, when new stirrings within begin to overwhelm and physical changes can be felt, and observed by others, and yet go unexplained. Such anxiety created, in the main, by ignorance affects learning in all areas of the curriculum in all forms of education and can be particularly noticeable in standards in examinable

81

subjects. This is true of highly intelligent pupils as well as the average and less academically able.

Anxiety is probably most often created when the individual feels himself to be different from his peer group. Yet this is bound to be a common occurrence because of the wide age span covered by adolescence. One boy's growth spurt may start at twelve years and he will tower above his contemporaries with his broader shoulders, deep voice and more manly appearance. His friend may well commence his period of rapid growth at fifteen and for what will seem an eternity to the smaller boy, he will appear childish, unformed and incomplete by comparison. Similarly the girl who feels lumpy with developed breasts and broadening hips feels odd if her peers are lightly turning somersaults or standing on their hands upside down against a school wall. The slow developing girl feels inadequate for contrary reasons. Such feelings of inadequacy and insecurity undermine confidence and hamper a buoyant approach to life. It can diminish curiosity and the drive to learn. It probably also saps vitality unnecessarily.

Our knowledge of the difficulties of adolescents, derived from the research of Schofield and of others who have worked with young people, shows us that we have a responsibility to give information and begin to talk with young people about future development at a time when this is relevant to interest and before adolescent feelings are very strong. A gentle and sensitive approach which takes into account the growing awareness of the beginnings of adolescent change can again be made in many ways according to the themes current in the general learning or the teacher's own particular interests. Early learning is likely to be incidental but there will come a time, as in the story about babies and birth, when it is appropriate to bring items of related knowledge together.

The radiovision strip 'Growing Up', with its accompanying tape, is just such a sensitive and child-centred approach to this. The drawings are by Sheila Bewley as were those of 'Where Do Babies Come From?' and the style is the same. Its aim is to prepare boys and girls for the feelings they will have, and some are beginning to have, and the physical changes they will observe in themselves and others by ensuring that they have the facts to come to an understanding of what is happening to themselves and their fellows. It builds on the theory given in 'Where Do Babies Come

From?' and the 'Merry-Go-Round' programmes and particularly enlarges on the information touched on in the last programme, 'Full Circle'. Here there was a brief mention of menstruation in the context of fertilisation followed by cell division. In 'Growing Up' this knowledge is given in the context of reproduction as being an essential condition for a new life to start and also in a personal practical way as a part of normal growing up which is most constructive and helpful.

Information on boys' development includes circumcision but excludes seminal emission or 'wet dreams'. It is likely that this could be included in any modified version which is made, particularly if teachers inform the BBC educational officers that they think this would be valuable. It is something which often arises in discussions but which the writer believes it would be wise to include in the story of 'Growing Up' itself, as some boys may hesitate to ask for what they want to know if they feel the invitation to ask is not sufficiently explicit. From this it may sometimes be appropriate to convey sensitively that masturbation is a common way of releasing feelings. This is not likely to be explored in much detail at this stage, but an acknowledgement by the teacher is likely to be reassuring and the word itself may have been used so that a question can be more easily framed at a stage which requires more information or reassurance.

As boys and girls normally learn together in most junior classes or groups it will be an accepted arrangement for this learning too. At a stage when emotional feelings are not overwhelming there is likely to be enormous benefit in boys beginning to learn something about the changes in girls, and girls learning about the changes in boys. Further theory given in the adolescent years in secondary schools may well be better given separately, although at about fifteen to seventeen years and beyond, learning together again seems best particularly in discussion of aesthetic and moral concepts and a deeper understanding of personal feelings and human relationships.

In these years, when co-education is normal, it seems wise to introduce boys as well as girls to menstruation in a factual and yet sensitive way before either are personally involved. From such knowledge of reality greater consideration of one half of the human race for the other half is likely to be incorporated and developed. Teachers who can bring in facts about seminal emission, even though at present excluded in the radiovision strip itself, could also ensure a similar understanding of boys by girls which could contribute at a later stage to an understanding of the physical sexual drive and quick arousal in men compared with women. This latter piece of specific information will be inappropriate at this early stage but such information as is appropriate, namely seminal emission, is likely to contribute to a growing awareness and understanding at a later stage.

The story of 'Growing Up' repeats the very important message for these years that everyone is different and grows up at a different rate. It also restates the view expressed in 'Full Circle' that human beings have a great deal to find out and that, even when we believe we have grown up, we find we still have a great deal more to learn. This seems to most of us a wise idea for young people to consider seriously and discuss.

Here is the commentary broadcast on BBC1 in the Nature Series for use with the radiovision strip. This is given in Notes for Teachers N257 and is obtainable from BBC. The notes in italics are not part of the commentary itself but are included in the notes.

'Growing Up' Commentary
Title Frame
This is BBC Radio 4 for schools. 'Nature'—'Growing Up'. This radiovision broadcast is accompanied by a filmstrip, teachers' notes and pamphlets for the children.
'Growing Up'. You should be looking at the title frame of the filmstrip now. After the speaker has finished describing each frame there will be about 10 seconds of music, then a brief pause. Turn to the next frame when the music stops. But turn to the first frame now.

1. New born baby.
Hello. Do you remember what it was like being a baby? I don't suppose you do. This is a new baby about a week old. You probably looked like this when you were born, with a rather wrinkly face, tiny hands and feet, and a navel that sticks out a bit.
Before birth a baby has been growing at a very fast rate, from an egg the size of a pencil dot to a human being about 20 inches long and $7\frac{1}{2}$ pounds weight. After birth the growth rate decreases. If it didn't, we'd be taller than Nelson's column at the age of seventy.

2. Breast feeding.

Babies drink milk as their first food, either from their mother's breast, as you see here, or from a bottle. At first a baby has to be fed every few hours, night and day. But after a few months it has meals more or less at the same time as the rest of the family.

Human milk is sweeter and more dilute than cow's milk, and is the best food for the first few weeks of life. A baby's weight generally increases at the rate of about 6–8 oz. a week during the first six months.

3. Children and mother.

Growing up is a long job. It takes years to grow up to be an adult human being. It usually takes about a whole year before a baby can even stand up on its own feet. In this picture the baby is just learning to crawl. The girl is older, about two years old, and she can walk quite well. Children depend on their parents for a far greater proportion of their life span than the offspring of other mammals.

4. Boy.

This boy is about eight years old and he is already quite grown-up when you compare him to the children in the last picture. His body is more in the shape of a man, not nearly so round as it was as a baby. It takes a long time to learn all the things a grown-up has to know.

How the proportions of the body change during childhood is illustrated in the pupils' pamphlet.

5. Girl.

This girl is about eight years old too, and, like the boy, she's a slimmer and taller shape than she was as a baby. And she knows a lot too, just like the boy. But there's still a lot of growing up and learning to happen, to both the girl and the boy. Let's talk about girls first.

6. Older girl.

One of the first things that happens to the girl in the next stage of growing up is that her breasts develop. All women have breasts. They can begin to grow quite early, at about nine or so, or they may not show until later, say fourteen or fifteen. It doesn't matter how soon or late they come. Everybody is different and grows up at a different rate. This girl is wearing a bra which is a good idea because it feels comfortable.

The average age of the beginning of breast development is before the eleventh birthday, but as with all aspects of puberty, the range of ages is wide, in this case from nine years to fourteen or fifteen years, and it is absolutely normal for breasts to begin to develop at any time within this range.

7. Female anatomy.

Another thing that happens to girls as they grow up is that their insides begin to work like a woman's. If you could see inside a woman's body it would look something like this. In the picture you can see the bones of the hip and, in the middle, the womb. That's the pink triangular part. The two parts at the sides of the womb are the ovaries where all the eggs are kept. A girl is born with thousands of undeveloped eggs in each ovary. As she grows up some of these eggs develop and, every four weeks, one minute egg travels from one of the ovaries to the womb.

And every four weeks a smooth lining develops inside the womb. If the egg gets fertilised by sperm from a man, it attaches itself to the lining and grows into a baby. If it does not get fertilised it breaks up, and together with the lining it comes out, with some blood, through the vagina. All girls have periods like this from about eleven or twelve, but like growing breasts, everyone is different and some girls may start earlier and some much later. *The first menstrual period is known as the menarche. The menarche is usually the last of the pubertal changes for girls, coming after breast development, pubic hair, the general rounding out of the contours and towards the end of the growth spurt referred to in the introduction which last is of great psychological importance to the adolescent. It can be quite consoling for a girl to know that, as her first period comes, she is likely to have finished growing at the increased rate. The average age for the menarche is now about thirteen but it is quite normal for it to happen at any age between eleven and fifteen.*

8. Woman with sanitary pad.

Periods happen about every four weeks and they last for three or four days. They don't hurt, and girls very soon get used to having them. The only thing is, you have to wear a small, soft, cotton-wool pad when you're having a period, so that the blood doesn't mark your clothes. They're called sanitary pads or towels. This one is attached to a thin elastic band that goes round the waist. The pads are quite small and neat and you can't tell that a girl is wearing one when her clothes are on as well.

Periods are most irregular at the beginning and end of a woman's fertile life, i.e. at adolescence and at the menopause. As well as the type of sanitary towel illustrated here there are other kinds, known as tampons, that are worn internally, i.e. within the vagina.

9. Pubic and underarm hair, female.

One more thing about girls before we go on to boys. About this time hair begins to grow on their bodies, both round the vagina and under the arms. All women have hair in these two places. It usually begins to grow at about the same time as the breasts begin to develop—at any time between the ages of nine and fifteen. But again, everybody's different, and grows up at a different rate.

It is quite normal for pubic hair to begin to grow at any age from nine to fifteen, and to be completely grown at any age from twelve to seventeen. The average age for it to begin growing is twelve, and for it to be completely grown, fifteen.

10. Boy's genitalia.

Boys' bodies change too, as they get older. Under the penis the boy has a little bag of skin with two round things like balls inside it. They are called testicles. From the age of eleven or so until old age the testicles produce sperm which a man needs to help make a baby grow inside a woman. The sperm comes up from the testicles into the penis and out of the tiny opening at the end.

Boys are born with penis and testicles but, unlike girls, where the ova are present in an undeveloped state from birth, a boy's sperm only begins to be made at puberty. Both penis and testicles begin to grow larger at any time between nine-and-a-half and thirteen-and-a-half. The average age for their development is eleven-and-a-half. Sperm begins to be produced at the same time. It either stays in the testicles, or is passed out during masturbation or during 'wet dreams'. Only a very small quantity of liquid is passed out at any time—about a teaspoonful.

11. Circumcised and uncircumcised penises.

When a boy is born he has a little bit of skin round the tip of the penis. Sometimes this little band of skin is taken off when he is a few days old—he is circumcised. The boy on the left has been circumcised, the boy on the right has not. Some boys are, some boys are not. Some parents and doctors think it is healthier if the skin is taken off and some don't. Both sorts of penis work perfectly well. The penis has two main uses: it's the tube that carries the sperm out of the man's body, and also the tube that carries the urine out when the man goes to the lavatory. The penis can't carry both liquids at the same time, so they never get mixed up. In young boys the penis really only has one use, for urine, because young boys don't have any sperm. It's only when boys grow up to be men that it has these two uses.

Circumcision is a matter of (a) religion and (b) medical fashion. The fashion varies from time to time and place to place. At the present moment medical opinion in London is rather against the automatic circumcision of baby boys as being unnecessary surgery.

12. Pubic, chest and underarm hair, male.
Another thing that happens to boys is that hair grows on their bodies, under the arms and low down on the body around the penis. But hair can also grow on their chests as you can see here. The hair around the penis can begin to grow at any time from about eleven to about fifteen. The hair on the chest comes much later. Some men don't ever have hair on their chests, some don't have much, and some have a lot.

13. Head of a boy.
A little bit later other changes happen to boys as they become young men. For one thing their vocal chords grow longer and they begin to speak with deep voices. In the weeks the chords are developing, the boy may speak partly in his old child's voice, and partly in his new man's voice. And it begins to show on the outside —he begins to have an Adam's apple. And hair begins to grow on boys' faces, on the chin and upper lip. At first this hair is soft and there isn't a great deal of it.

A longer length of string, when vibrated, will have a lower note than a shorter length. Thus long vocal chords make a voice sound deep. The voice change in boys comes slightly after the maximum growth rate, usually between the ages of twelve and sixteen.

14. Three faces.
The changes that we've been talking about go on all through the years from ten or eleven to about eighteen. During these years you are learning all the time, each year a little more, about what it's like to be a grown-up person. Even when you think you are quite grown-up at about seventeen or eighteen you'll find that there is still more to learn about growing up, and growing older.

It's a story that goes on and on, right through life from the beginning to the end.

The body is an organism that is continually changing. Before birth and during infancy, it develops very quickly. Changes are more gradual during the years of childhood up to puberty. At puberty, the growth rate accelerates to a pace comparable to that of infancy. Following puberty is a long period of adult life where ageing processes are at first very gradual. The fertile life of a woman stops somewhere around forty-five. Men can produce fertile sperm until their very old age. Men die, on average, at sixty-eight, women at seventy-four.

Credit frame.

That was a radiovision programme from the Nature Series, written by Margaret Sheffield and presented by Elizabeth Ornbo. The pictures in the filmstrips were by Sheila Bewley. The music was composed and played by Gilbert Biberian.

When children see 'Growing Up' they are reminded of 'Where Do Babies Come From?' and there is usually a request to see this again. This is an ideal opportunity for relearning but teachers will of course not be surprised if the questions require more detailed answers than those asked when learning took place earlier.

Much of the vocabulary will be already known but in case the following words have not been used in learning about babies, their growth and birth, they are listed here and should now be included as they are essential for understanding.

male	external genitalia penis	scrotum	testes (testis)
female	external genitalia labia	vagina	
puberty, breast	nipple	bra, brassiere	
body proportions			
ovaries, ovary	womb	uterus	
fertilised sperm	seminal fluid		
menstruation	menstrual period	menarche (first menstruation)	

pubic hair		underarm hair	facial hair
sanitary	sanitary pads, towels	tampons	
'wet dreams'		masturbation	
circumcised	circumcision		
urine	excreta		
vocal cords	Adam's apple	shave	beard
embryo	foetus	baby	infant toddler
adolescence	adolescent		
adult	mature	maturity	

The booklet gives the following suggestions for children's active learning and teachers will think of many others relevant to their own particular learning situations.

1. Weigh and measure the height of each child in the class. Graph the results. Is there any difference in the average weight and height of boys and girls? Repeat this weighing and measuring at three monthly intervals. Are the boys growing faster than the girls, or the girls faster than the boys?

2. Let the children use the pupils' pamphlet as a record book for their own development. On the back cover there are weight and height graphs which the children can fill in with their own measurements. However, be careful to emphasise that difference in individual body size at this stage is quite unimportant: little children may grow up to be big adults, and vice versa.

3. Work out methods of recording the growth rates of other parts of the body such as fingernails and hair.

4. Closely observe the changes from immature to adult in other animals, for instance in birds, frogs, ponies or cats. As appropriate, draw pictures, take or collect photographs, describe in words, weigh and measure, and try to record the growth rate graphically.

5. With older girls, say those of age 10 plus, it would be appropriate at some time to have a visitor from the Health Department to explain the practical details of coping with menstruation.

The following account of sex education in a school is by the headmistress of a one-form entry, mixed infant and junior school. It shows how the school has brought the subject into general learning in all sorts of incidental ways from the infant class upwards and how the knowledge learned incidentally is brought together with 'Where Do Babies Come From?' at about eight years of age and the 'Merry-Go-Round' series at about nine plus, with 'Growing Up' at ten and eleven with the use of 'Where Do Babies. Come From?' again. The infant classes are vertically grouped.

In our school the sex education programmes on TV and radiovision have been accepted as part of the school curriculum.

There are books and pamphlets at all levels of reading, for the children to read and ask questions.

Animals and fish are kept in the school and the children talk about the 'fat guppies' having babies. A baby guinea-pig arrived at school this week, brought by a child in a class where guinea-pigs are being cared for. There was class discussion about mating and growth. (Nine-year-old children.)

The infants have grown seeds (peas, beans, etc.) and at present stick insects are hatching at a rapid rate. This all has a bearing on spring and new growth. The children also went to see the new chicks and ducklings on the lake. Discussion and various forms of art work followed.

There is a pleasant relationship between parents and teachers, and parents report questions being asked at home —a boy while bathing asked 'Was I circumcised, Mummy?'

After seeing the films and holding discussions at the parent-teacher meeting, only one parent asked for a child (girl) to be withdrawn. I have respected the parent's wish and the child has been quietly given other things to do, but she has been present in class when children were asking questions, and the literature is available for all the children to read.

A member of this staff, a young man in his second year of teaching, used 'Merry-Go-Round' with his mainly nine-year-olds within an organisation which allowed for integrated study particularly in science and environmental work. He reports:

My general impression was that a great deal of thought and planning had gone into the series. It was logical in its presentation and encouraged a great deal of thought and discussion among the children.

The series was dovetailed into the normal curriculum. Before the first programme, we had discussions regarding baby animals and had carried out various physiological experiments, lung capacity, pulse rates, etc. As the series progressed we were able to carry out the follow-up suggestions, regarding body measurements, etc.

Most of the children were very settled during the programme, however there was a little embarrassment at certain shots. During the discussions which followed each session, the children asked a great many frank and sensible questions.

Various recommended publications were available, and on a number of occasions group discussion was initiated by various members of the class.

The headmistress joined this class for the last programme and follow-up work. This is a usual thing in this school where co-operation between head and staff is marked. She noted:

There was great interest and little embarrassment.
There was interest in twins—how they were formed. Identical twins in school were examined.
A double-yolk egg was brought to school by a boy who kept chickens. This was examined with particular interest.
Dissimilar twins were discussed.
Children's likeness to parents and grandparents, etc. Work on comparison continues.
One girl asked 'Can you marry your brother?'
Why do babies look like their parents?
I have no recollection of any questions from a boy regarding his own body and probably none concerning a girl's body, but then, in a mixed group discussion, the questions are answered for all.

The deputy head writes of his class work:

We used the radiovision programmes 'Where Do Babies Come From?' and 'Growing Up' with my ten and eleven-year-olds. They were used in conjunction with work on rebirth, spring, growth and Easter eggs last year. BBC series 'Science All Around' on reproduction of plants and creatures provided a good setting for this year.

Preparations. Books on birth and development of the human body were available and circulated among members of the class. (*Where Do Babies Come From?* by the National Marriage Guidance Council I have found particularly valuable.) Opportunities were taken for drawing attention to physical reproduction in nature. Relationships both of respect and of love between people were emphasised.

Presentation. The broadcasts were shown in the school hall to the whole class of thirty-five, in a calm quiet period of the day. The filmstrip 'Where Do Babies Come From?' was shown both this year and last to the older children, as they had not previously had the opportunity to see it, and because of the high turnover of children in our school which meant that many had not seen it. The commentary was too simple for the age seeing it and the notes had to be adapted and read, rather than the tape used directly. The simplicity of the presentation on tape was lost, but the commentary was more suitable to the age of the children. It might be possible to combine the two methods in some way, next time.

'Growing Up' was shown a few days after 'Where Do Babies Come From?' and the radiovision programme used in its entirety. Whilst watching 'Where Do Babies Come From?' there was the occasional nervous laugh from one boy, but 'Growing Up' was listened to in silence and with concentration. The programme was undertaken in a 'cool' manner as a normal part of the term's work.

Follow-up. Children were happy to discuss the programme in informal situations, and to initiate discussions of quite specific matters—and they were given the opportunity to record their impressions but in very few cases took this up. Informal conversations after the showing suggested that the programme confirmed what was already known from books, from parents, etc. Few admitted to even the slightest embarrassment and only one showed signs by turning her eyes away from the screen on one or two occasions.

I believe that to require specific work to be produced from the series would be an improper intrusion into their privacy. The learning continues in conversation and reading and in the maturing of their personalities.

I noted down these questions which followed the two radiovision programmes. They were nearly all framed for confirmation of what was viewed and read. Girls' questions seemed to me to be of a personal nature:

'Is it true that tampons can get lost inside?'

'Do schools hold stocks of sanitary towels for emergencies?'

'Does a girl's ability in sports suffer when she's having a period?'

'Why are women more bad-tempered when having a period?'

'How does the sperm get to the egg?'

'What happens if a lot of sperm reaches them at once?'

'What happens to the sperm which don't reach the egg?'

'What happens to the egg which is not fertilised?'

'Has a girl all the eggs in her body when she is born?'

'How can girls of nine and ten have a baby?'

'Is it painful to have a baby?'

'Why is a pregnant mother sick in the mornings?'

'Why can't some mothers have babies?'

(After the recent multiple births in Australia and elsewhere.)

Boy's questions seem to differ in that they enquire rather from curiosity than personal involvement.

'Won't we have test-tube babies in the future to save the mother from discomfort?'

'What are identical twins?'

'What are Siamese twins?'

'What are blue babies?'

'Does it hurt to have a baby?'

The headmaster of another infant and junior school sees his way very clearly in this area of learning and has had his own particular approach established for some years. He is a most experienced head who is well known to parents and trusted by them in all educational matters. He believes that a formal body of knowledge should be given in the third and fourth junior school years. He is a teaching head and he writes:

As you know I am not happy with the idea of a sex education programme geared for primary pupils below the last year . . .

and certainly would express an objection to any suggestion that children should be confronted with filmstrips and films and broadcasts without a series of thorough in-class discussions and preparation. This latter comment also applies, as far as I am concerned, with my ten- and eleven-year-old pupils, having found over the years—and well before the BBC programmes—that such a delicate subject should be approached only when there is that indefinable rapport between a class and their teacher . . . Mutual confidence, coupled with mutually sympathetic respect, seems to me essential.

To many people, the connotations underlying the unfortunate term 'Sex Education' are arbitrarily misleading. I endeavour to avoid it as much as possible; I have perforce to use the word 'sex' to the children but I prefer to use the umbrella-term, 'The Story of You!' and so cunningly exploiting their unashamed self-interest! This makes them sit up—or is it 'down' these days?—and listen, talk, question and pour out their hearts. They are truly fascinated by the boomerang comments but do let me emphasise that they never know when comes the next instalment of 'The Story'; so that they cannot say: 'Oh yes, we *do* sex education third period on a Thursday morning' . . . I remember—and hope they do—the Last Instalment and only when the opportunity arises do I continue the serial and, of course, the opportunities for re-introduction and continuity in top-class juniors are legion—for example: The first Brimstone in March; the Birth of Jesus—and of Caesar; the binary scale in their Dads' scientific work at AERE; the queried life on Mars, in their simple observational astronomy; characteristics of past invaders of our country (a glorious opportunity for the introduction of genes!); love of grandparents, noticeably maternal; pets, pets and more pets; the village racehorse-training stables and stud; the local Agricultural Research Centre, to witness the stages in breeding of small animals; the local midwife's popularity and her busy non-seasonal life; gestation and graph work; the pupils' own doctors; graphs of their places—and countries—of birth; maternity fashions (ostensibly for the girls—although the boys knowingly smile when I sketch one); their waxing interest in pop-music; the school's cardinal sin of Litter (leading to public Graffiti—which they all have seen anyway); a particular family, including a single, twins and triplets; the stone curlew's immemorial spring return to the Downs—yes, the opportunities are infinite.

My 'Story' lasts from September to June, when we culminate nowadays, after much *repeated* discussion, with the BBC 'Merry-Go-Round' films . . . but please do not think that the theme is overplayed—on the contrary, as one can see by the opportunities listed, it is thoughtfully woven into the delightful web of their life, exploiting that sense of wonder of the World-So-Old-And-All.

They are instructed (unashamedly does he use that emotive word) in the elementary physiology of sex, quite objectively before the inevitable onset of the emotional associations. The naturalness is emphasised and at the same time their curiosity is stimulated, making them question me, question each other, their relatives, their parents—most do with their parents, but a few never do, especially if they, like their teacher, have had Welsh nonconformist genes handed down!

I am happy in the thought that they will enter their secondary phase at least theoretically well-equipped and secure in their own *true* knowledge . . . knowing the basic facts of 'The Story', so that although they may have occasion to refer furtively to the family medical dictionary or to the Song of Solomon and will have secret conversations with friends—they will not be frightened by alarming stories creatively told by unpleasant—or insecure—older children.

Without question, a prerequisite is the willing agreement of their parents, Dad noticeably being pleased that teacher will cover a subject which can be unconscionably embarrassing to him . . . In the years I have been telling 'The Story of You', I have not yet had a dissident Dad or a vetoing Mum—but I am fortunate in that I am *known* (for better or worse) by the populace.

I cannot really send you a curricular plan as it depends on the episode reached but I usually take a traditional approach, starting with the evolutionary approach (here, I believe, top juniors can just about appreciate the comparison with the religious origin)—then, the usual development of fish, amphibia, reptiles, monsters, etc. (and useful here, the school's accumulated and mounted collection of graptolites, trilobites, crinoids, ammonites, mammoth teeth, sharks' teeth, dinosaurs' vertebrae, etc.). From there to the girl's body (preferably first), to the boy's body, woman's, man's— then human egg and sperm (an interested local doctor arranges pathological slides)—the growth of baby in the womb (having described, in the words of E. R. Matthews, the sexual act so simply—but repeated and repeated in different ways as some pupils, I am sure, do not really believe it!)— the birth of the baby—and always, emphasis on the happy secure love-relationship of the parents.

My pupils do not, in my opinion, require much practical work such as casting wombs and embryos in clay—fortunately I sketch reasonably—and parents have prepared permanent displays, suitably mounted, for the children's use . . . and we do no written work as I want to keep this peripheral—hence the long series—as I do not want to over-emphasise.

Most years I am fortunate in recruiting a real baby-rearing Mum to talk to the class (from early to pre-natal pregnancy); she is measured, weighed and questioned—and with no little awe.

E. R. Matthews I, and parents, think delightful, undramatic and more than adequate and the children use it, as they do other books on the county list.

. . . I do hope that this has not appeared too sketchy but I believe that all salient points have been covered.

I feel I must repeat that, although teachers should answer honestly any question by a child up to the age of nine, I personally would not tell such children 'The Story of You' as I am not *quite* sure if they are ready; I often wonder if I am over-sentimental in wanting them to keep for as long as possible their native innocence? And secondly, I believe that 'The Story'—in depth—should only be explored when there exists a near-ideal rapport between the teacher and the children.

Types of questions parents ask:
'Will the whole story be told?'
'Does the word 'love' come into it?'
'Have you seen any apparent distress?'

'Do the children ask questions?'
'What books would you recommend?'
'Do you mention poor Dad as well as Mum?'

Chapter 6

Questions often asked by children

Children's questions show a fairly common pattern and can be roughly classified into three kinds. There are questions which arise when parts of the story are not sufficiently clear to enable understanding to be commensurate with interest. There are questions related to old wives' tales and bizarre ideas and a seeking for a truthful interpretation or explanation of them. There are questions which relate to moral aspects of the theory.

Very many teachers in today's primary schools will be accustomed to coping with children's questions on all manner of topics. They will answer directly if they know the answer or introduce the child to a source of information to answer the question for himself. They will also know that they sometimes have to say that they don't know the answer but will find out. It is just as appropriate to approach questions in this area of knowledge in this manner as in any other. It is quite likely that a question will be posed to which a teacher won't immediately have the answer, for we are not so accustomed to working with children in this area as in some others and have a less clear idea of their interests in this. With experience it will become easier and easier to meet children's needs and answer questions. Indeed, as most of the questions are asked by most children, we shall have the answers ready.

However, from experience of working with children in other topics it is possible to have an idea of an individual child's mode of questioning and to anticipate some questions and the child or children who will be most forward in formulating them. On the other hand, one should not allow oneself to be surprised by an unexpected question but bear in mind that there is nothing wrong in needing to stand still and think about a question for a minute. Children who are used to informal ways of working with a teacher will be used to this kind of partnership in thinking and planning. We do know that there is a correlation between a thinking teacher and the thinking of the children who work with her.

In all areas of the curriculum teachers are accustomed to reading up and finding out for themselves the facts and background to the topics which are being currently studied. The books in Appendix B are primarily for fairly able children and will give teachers the sort of information children want to have. Books in Appendix C are for adults and offer suggestions on approaches and also some background on the thinking behind practice in education in general and sex education in particular.

To meet children's intellectual and emotional needs at primary-middle school level it is not necessary for a teacher to study medical tomes, embryology, theories of inheritance and Mendel and Darwin, etc. We do not need specialist teachers. It is likely that this will be found to be interesting reading if not already known, but, in the years we are considering, it is the relevance to self which is important and therefore it is the human aspects which mostly arouse curiosity and interest. The aim is to give an accurate basic outline on which detailed scientific medical theory can be added commensurate with ability and interest. Specifically it is to give the story of human beings which enables a child to grow emotionally as well as intellectually into an understanding of human behaviour and drives, and from this to arrive at a code of personal principles and behaviour in relation to the facts.

As was mentioned in Chapter 1 it is wise to accept the principle that if a child is able to frame a question he has sufficient insight to have some idea of what the answer will be. He has partial knowledge. It could perhaps be said that a teacher's success in any part of the curriculum could be measured, in some respects, by how often she arouses curiosity to motivate learning and then maintains curiosity so that the desire for further knowledge is shown by a questioning approach.

Questions which require theory of any depth and hence specialist knowledge are not usually asked in the middle school and upper junior school years. Questions are largely personal and concerned with a collection of simple facts and with getting the outline straight, the sequence of events in order. Questions will be repeated over the years and repetition of nearly the same answer from teachers, parents and other adults is likely to confirm learning. Children tend to check up on us.

Questions are still egocentrically slanted at about eight to eleven. The largest number still tend to be about the baby and the child takes the answers to fill out his knowledge of himself. Children usually ask questions about the egg or ovum, the beginning of the baby,

> e.g. How big is the egg, ovum?
>
> How does it get inside the mother's tummy, uterus?
>
> How does it stay in the uterus and not fall out?

Some of these questions, for instance, the size of the ovum, will be answered incidentally earlier in the infant or first school as we become accustomed to incorporating this knowledge into general learning though the questions may continue to be asked later.

The following basic facts will probably give most junior/middle school children what they want to know. A few within this age range who want more detail are likely to be the ones who can supplement the facts given orally with those obtained from books. Nevertheless a teacher will find out what is needed for this stage too without difficulty. Conversely some nine- and ten-year-olds may not want all this detail and a sensitive teacher will assess the degree needed as the questioning and talking proceeds.

1. It is better to use the term 'ovum' as soon as possible and drop the term 'egg' as soon as the carry-over in thinking from egg to ovum has started. It may be necessary with some children to state quite categorically that the ovum is not a bit like the egg we eat for breakfast.

2. Similarly 'sperm' should be used and not 'seed'. The fact that a teaspoonful of semen contains millions of sperm is interesting to fact collectors.

3. The ovum is smaller than a full stop or a grain of granulated sugar or a grain of sand. We can just see it without needing a

microscope or magnifying glass if we have sharp eyes. A single sperm is so small that we cannot see it without a microscope. Each ovary—there are two—is about as big as a grape, or the end part of a grown-up's finger or your big toe. The uterus is about as big as your closed fist.

4. All baby girls are born with millions of undeveloped ova in their ovaries. They are stored safely in the ovaries until a girl reaches menarche. Menarche is the name we give to a stage in growing when a girl is nearly grown up, nearly a young woman.

A large but simple diagram drawn on a blackboard or other writing surface if the teacher is skilful will be valuable. A diagram on card prepared beforehand by the less skilful is just as good if the teacher explains it fully to each new set of pupils. Simple diagrams are in *Growing Up*, Book 4, *Right from the Start* and relevant BBC Pupils' Pamphlets. Young children cannot always understand enlarged diagrams of internal organs if the outline body shape, which they know, is not included.

At menarche one ovum leaves one ovary and this continues periodically. This period is usually about twenty-eight days. The ovum leaves the right ovary at one period and then the left the next period and this continues alternately. The ovum moves along the fallopian tube. If a sperm reaches the ovum and fertilises it as it moves along the fallopian tube to the uterus the ovum and sperm join together and then begin to divide into two cells, then four, then eight, and so on. The growing ovum attaches itself to the lining of the uterus and continues to grow into a baby.

This forms most of the story of conception within menstruation. If the question has been about the beginning of a baby growing, one stops here but shows one will go on if more is wanted. If the question is more specifically on menstruation, for example,

Why do women have to have a period before they can have a baby?

Do all girls have periods?

Do animals have periods as well as humans?

How can you tell when you are going to have a period?

When a girl or lady has a period how much blood comes out? then the rest of the cycle can be added—that if a sperm does not meet the ovum and fertilise it, the ovum does not begin to grow by cell division. It does not attach itself to the uterus and grow into a baby. It moves to the uterus but does not stay there. The uterus is lined with blood to be ready for a fertilised ovum. If the ovum is not fertilised by a sperm it passes down out of the vagina with the blood from the uterus. This is called menstruation or having a period.

All girls when they begin to be young women menstruate or have a period about every twenty-eight days. When all the blood has passed out—this takes about three or four days—the uterus begins to build up a new supply of blood in case the next ovum released from the ovary on the opposite side is fertilised and needs to attach itself to the blood supply in the uterus. This carries on in a cycle over and over again. One of the indications which a mother has that she may be going to have a baby is when she does not have a period or does not menstruate.

5. Girls begin to menstruate at about ten or eleven or twelve or thirteen or fourteen, fifteen or even seventeen. Each girl is different and it doesn't matter at what age periods start. All are usually quite normal.

6. Menstruation goes on in a fairly regular cycle until about the age of forty-five to forty-nine years. That is why we notice that older women do not usually have babies.

At about eight and nine years the details and practicalities of menstruation may not be wanted, as it is less relevant than it will become later. At ten to eleven years, however, the practical side of menstruation is needed. It is nicely explained in 'Growing Up' and the inclusion of the filmstrip provides a sound and helpful approach to which further detail can be added by the teacher as it is needed.

In talking about menstruation it seems wise to suggest that most girls and women take the cycle of menstruation in their stride for this is likely to assist the development of an embracing, on-going attitude to life in girls themselves. We know of occasional cases of women who suffer acute menstrual discomfort but we also know that in these cases there is often an element of apprehension, anticipation of pain, a creation of tension derived from attitudes to menstruation engendered in the early years.

Knowledge of ovulation and menstruation often now brings questions on the pill from older junior school and middle school children which reveal the snippets of information they glean from adult conversation and mass communication. It is interesting to notice how their questions are most often asked when the relevant part of the story is reached. Some questions on this aspect are:

1. Does a mother have a certain amount of children?
2. How many children can she have?
3. Why can't older women have children?
4. How do you stop having babies? Do you have to take pills?
5. If a lady took the pill, could she have another baby after?

To our knowledge the only method of contraception mentioned by children is the pill though Chanter in his book shows that a boy had some idea of a condom as he knew the word, Durex.

The sort of information which answers the first three questions has been outlined above. To answer the fourth I suggest one gives information about the pill because there is already partial knowledge. One should be honest in acknowledging that there are other methods if one is asked though to suggest that this information will be more easily understood when they are older is probably enough. The following points could be conveyed:

i) From very early times men and women have sometimes wished that they need only have the children that they wanted to have and which they could look after properly. Men and women have discovered different ways to do this. A modern scientific way is for the mother to take a pill which affects her cycle of menstruation (producing an ovum each period). Simply put, the pill makes the body behave as though the mother is pregnant when no ovum is produced so it is not there to be fertilised by a sperm and grow into a baby. If there is no ovum there cannot be a baby.

ii) One could say that the name given to ways of preventing a baby growing is called contraception—against conception.

Another set of questions on the baby relates to the next stage in development of the foetus. They are mostly concerned with the umbilical cord and nourishment of the baby.

How does the baby feed inside the mother?

How does the baby breathe inside the mother?

A child often finds it difficult to comprehend that all the mother eats, e.g. bacon and egg for breakfast, doesn't pass straight down in this form through the umbilical cord to the baby as it passes down his own oesophagus. It is difficult to explain this satisfactorily and it is wise to say that this is a very complicated process and that they will be able to understand better when they learn more biology later on. However, it is necessary to try to give an accurate basis for future theory which helps understanding at this stage. One could establish these points:

1. The mother digests the food for herself and the baby. All digested food is liquid. (A topic on digestion covered earlier will help understanding as in Nelson's *Growing Up*, Book 2. *The Human Body*, Puffin Book 102. *Your Body*, Ladybird, Wills & Hepworth.)

2. The umbilical cord attaches the baby by his middle to a part of his mother's uterus called the placenta.

3. Mother's blood circulates through blood vessels like tiny tubes round her body including the placenta.

4. Baby's blood circulates round its body in blood vessels including the umbilical cord.

5. The mother's blood is separate from the baby's blood, in the mother's blood vessels.

6. The baby's blood is separate from the mother's blood, in the baby's blood vessels.

7. The blood vessels are close together in the placenta. The walls of the blood vessels are thin. A special kind of liquid food passes through the thin walls from the mother's blood into the baby's blood. Waste from the baby's blood passes into the mother's blood and is passed out by the mother.

8. Oxygen is passed from the mother's blood to the baby's blood.

9. A baby does not breathe air with his lungs inside his mother. There is no air in the uterus. He uses his lungs to breathe with as soon as he is born. He nearly always cries and to do this he has to fill his lungs with air. A baby's first cry makes him start breathing and he goes on doing this all his life. When we are dead we have stopped breathing.

Children are interested in their own navels. It is evidence which supports the facts. The knowledge that they were once joined to their mother by their umbilical cord to the navel seems to give some children marked satisfaction.

Other common questions on the baby *in utero* are:

Does a baby smell things?

Does a baby hear?

Does a baby see?

These can be quite simply answered with 'NO'. The baby is able to do all these things as soon as he is born and has cried and started to breathe and live. Additional information on a baby's sight and focusing, etc. could perhaps be found out by a boy or girl with a new-born baby at home or by having a new baby in school for a little while.

Questions about birth itself are usually less numerous than those about the growth of the baby. Here are some examples:

Does it hurt a baby when it is born?

Does it hurt a mother when a baby is born?

How does the vagina stretch to let a baby out?

These points may help to answer these and similar questions quite simply:

1. It doesn't hurt a baby to be born.

2. At times it does hurt a mother when a baby is being born as in birth muscles are being used which are not often used. It is a different sort of pain from any other pain, however, because it is a useful pain and a necessary pain and a mother knows that soon she will have the baby for which she has waited for at least nine months. Most mothers forget all about the pain as soon as they have their baby. Most mothers think this pain is worth while. Some mothers don't have much pain at all. Usually the pain is less for babies born after the first one as muscles have done the pushing job before. Doctors and nurses help mothers.

3. The vagina is specially made to stretch when a baby is ready to be born. It stretches very slowly a little at a time. Babies take quite a long time to be born so that there is time for the vagina to stretch slowly and be ready. The 'Merry-Go-Round' analogy in 'Birth' of a rubber band round the fingers stretching and then contracting is a useful one and the children could try this for themselves:

Questions about a baby's sex are frequently asked, for example:

Does a mother know whether she will have a boy or a girl?

Can you choose to have a boy baby or a girl baby?

Can a doctor tell whether a mother is going to have a boy or a girl before it is born?

A straightforward answer could be that recently doctors and scientists have discovered a way of diagnosing the sex of an embryo. It is a complicated process and is likely to be used to check whether a baby is growing properly if the doctors suspect that something could be wrong. Normally it is unlikely to be used to find out the sex of an embryo because it is expensive and complicated and would not serve any useful purpose. We cannot change the sex of a baby. A mother knows the sex of her baby as soon as it is born and to know earlier cannot really be helpful in normal circumstances.

Sometimes one might sense that it could be wise to state that some mothers and fathers think they might want a boy, or perhaps a girl, but that when their own baby, made from a part of each of them, is actually born they invariably love the baby even if it is not the sex they thought they wanted. As we cannot choose to have a boy or a girl it is wise to remember this and then the birth of the baby is a nice surprise, like a birthday present can be.

Older juniors at about ten and eleven years may be interested in simple hereditary factors which can be best explained with a simple diagram or simply with pin figures.

With reference to the male and female figures the simple information could be given that the nucleus of each cell contains thread-like shapes called chromosomes which carry certain characteristics like hair colour, eye colour, skin colour, curly or straight hair, blood group, and certain abilities, etc. All ova carry a factor we call x and sperm carry either an x factor or a y factor. These factors determine the sex of a baby. As soon as the sperm from the father fertilises the ovum of the mother the sex of the baby is decided. If an ovum with x chromosomes from the mother is fertilised by a sperm with an x chromosome from the father, the baby has 2x chromosomes and is a girl. If the ovum with x chromosomes from the mother is fertilised by a sperm with y chromosomes from the father, the baby is a boy with x and y chromosomes. That means that the sex of a baby is determined by the sperm of the father. Some sperm carry a factor which starts a baby girl growing and some a factor which starts a baby boy growing.

An occasional question concerns premature babies and this can be answered with a simple explanation that sometimes a baby is born before it is fully grown at nine months and then it is usually smaller and lighter than full-term babies and has to be specially cared for. Hospitals have units for premature babies and if they are very small they may be kept in incubators which are free of germs and always kept at the right temperature until the babies grow strong enough to be taken home by their mothers.

Children of primary school age always ask questions about twins. The answers may be clearly given under the headings:

1. Dissimilar twins
2. Identical twins
3. Siamese twins

for the questions invariably come in this order. They are best answered with reference to a simple, clear diagram of twins *in utero* as in *Right from the Start* and Jill Kenner's *Where Do Babies Come From?* A simple explanation using the illustration can cover these points.

1. Dissimilar twins are not common but they are the most common kind of twin. Occasionally the ovary releases two ova instead of the usual one ovum into the fallopian tube and as there are millions of sperm released at a time into the vagina it is as easy for two ova to be fertilised by sperm as one.

   The fertilised ova attach themselves to a different part of the uterus and grow their own placenta and own umbilical cord. They grow in their own sac of water. They develop in just the same way as one ovum on its own. The only difference is that each baby is usually smaller and lighter in weight than when just one baby is growing in the uterus alone. The baby which is lying lower in the uterus is usually born first and after a while the second follows. They are different from each other (dissimilar) because each grew from a different ovum from the mother and a different sperm from the father.

2. Identical twins are very unusual. They start to grow when one ovum is fertilised by one sperm and then in dividing into two the two cells become separate and continue to grow into two identical babies. They are identical because they develop from the same sperm from the father and the same ovum from ther mother. They attach themselves to the same part of the uterus and share the same placenta but each is attached by its own umbilical cord from the navel. The baby which lies nearer to the vagina is nearly always born first and the second a little while later.

3. Siamese twins are very, very unusual. They are identical twins formed from one fertilised ovum which has nearly split into two but not quite and the embryos grow into two babies which are partly joined together, sometimes by a limb, sometimes by the head and sometimes by the spine.

Doctors look after the mother and the twins, which they separate after birth by a special operation if it is possible. This is a very unusual occurrence and so may be announced as news on television or in the newspapers which is why we hear about them but very rarely see such twins.

It may be that some children today will have overheard adult conversation and news reports on abortion, and older juniors may have partly comprehended this and want some verification. It is suggested that it is important to be truthful and acknowledge that abortion exists but a simple explanation something like this is all that is likely to be understood:— that sometimes for special reasons, perhaps for instance that a pregnant mother has had German measles and the baby could therefore be deformed, a mother asks a doctor to perform an operation to remove the foetus so that she is no longer pregnant. This is called abortion and can usually only be done when the foetus is very tiny and has not reached the stage of being like a baby.

I believe that most teachers will want to say that this is a very serious decision for a mother and father and doctor to have to make. Like contraception it is a difficult subject to explain with simplicity and yet accuracy for this age. Children however sense the moral implications inherent in this kind of decision-making, and the teacher who can suggest that when they are older they will want to know more about this and other matters and think about them is confirming their own half-formed ideas about their position and helping them to accept that learning and understanding grows as we grow.

The question 'Do you have to be married to have a baby?' can be answered with reference to theory, with recapitulation of the story of intercourse, conception and cell division. The question can then be put back to the children so that they think it out again and come to understand for themselves that for fertilisation to take place the scientific fact is that a man and a woman must be involved and that they do not have to be married. Marriage is not a scientific arrangement. It is an arrangement made by men and women for good reasons. As in answering the question on abortion, it is important to help children to think out why men and women usually marry before having a family. Questions to the children such as 'Why do you think men and women marry before becoming parents?' 'Do you think it is good for a baby to have only a mother?' help them to think about the subject and ideas for themselves and then discuss them with teachers and parents. If the time is opportune, a discussion about care of babies and mothers, all the attention babies need, what mothers and fathers do for their children, etc., will help them to consider as fully as they can at this stage the importance of stable relationships, family life and homes. It seems wise to suggest that they will want to think and talk about all these things when they are older. Parallel studies in religious education could link most relevantly with this.

Most teachers recognise that if they prepare themselves adequately for this area of learning they will be able to give children the theory which their level of understanding and maturation require. They will be able to meet children's needs in terms of factual knowledge. Sometimes they feel less secure in meeting children's needs in answering questions which have moral implications. Firstly, perhaps, we should remind ourselves that detailed moral answers are not usually understood at this age and that the most potent moral influence is the example of parents and other adults with whom children associate and whom they admire. Nevertheless children are usually seeking for a simple statement which confirms a nearly black and white view of life, and one is wise to preface an answer with 'Most people think, believe . . . ' and state too that we all have to think out what we believe is right now and when we are older. It seems to us that we must be truthful and non-evasive with children and that at the same time we should not burden them with moral ideas beyond their level of understanding. Children who know themselves to be illegitimate or who have sisters who have illegitimate children need to be helped to think about moral issues for themselves without this being too closely linked to their own circumstances. Often, therefore, where one has such children in one's class, a simple answer at the time is probably best followed by a more general approach on another occasion.

Some teachers have been worried that children will embarrass them by asking personal questions; questions which in normal situations would be an infringement of privacy and discourteous. To answer this, I believe we are back to relationships and the values and attitudes which are prevalent in the school. In a school with sound relationships children will not be insensitive to a teacher's feelings, and consideration for others, including teachers, will be normal.

Some questions may, at first, sound clumsy, perhaps over-direct, but experienced teachers will appreciate that direct, simple questioning is typical of children at this stage and that the questions are probably only appearing to be over-direct because the subject is new and we are unaccustomed to hearing children's questions on it. Indeed in our experience teachers have enjoyed answering children's questions because they have revealed their deep interest and they have formed part of a piece of total learning to which teacher and children have become fully committed.

Although it is not within our experience, it is possible to visualise a situation where children might deliberately wish to embarrass a teacher by asking a discourteous personal question. This will certainly be done intentionally and knowingly. There will be a reason for this and I suggest that it is likely to be an act of retaliation arising from antagonism, perhaps in an over-authoritarian school or classroom. Such schools are unlikely to be ready to move into sensitive areas of the curriculum.

Chapter 7

Some suggestions on problems facing headteachers

A number of education authorities have made provision in their In-Service Training Programme for courses in sex education for their teachers. The courses have different titles: Education for Family Life, Health Education and Education in Personal Relationships. They are similar in approach and have, in a general sense, the same aims.

One authority, with an established programme for both secondary and primary schools, encourages heads and teachers to consider all aspects of this learning within the context of personal relationships. Three-day residential courses are offered to headmasters and headmistresses of primary schools, infant and junior schools. Following this, if the head wishes, the same type of course can be attended by the deputy or, in small schools, an experienced member of staff.

Most of the course time is spent in discussion in small peer groups of no more than eight members under the guidance of skilled tutors. From hours of discussion, with colleagues, on the whole field of human relationships, heads have derived, in individual and sometimes unique ways, something of value for themselves and for their own particular schools. Sometimes this may be an increased awareness of the complex network of relationships which exists in a school and the community it serves. It may be deeper understanding of the different levels of relationships or again a keener appreciation of the link between relationships and school ethos. Sometimes the gain cannot, and indeed need not, be defined.

Within this context of human relationships, and at an appropriate time, the group is invited to consider whether learning in the early years should include a gradual introduction to the facts about human birth, life and behaviour which, within a child-supporting, parent-supporting school, could contribute to development of personality and satisfy children's curiosity about an aspect of the real, everyday world in which we know they are interested at different stages in their development. There is no set time for this, there is no set programme of work, there is no persuasion or pressure. It is an important principle that each headmaster or headmistress is responsible for curriculum in this area, as in all others, and is free to make a professional decision in the light of the educational aims each has for his/her respective school.

The reason for offering these courses to headteachers first is based on a concept of the role of the headteacher, particularly at the primary, first and middle school level of education. This concept holds, among other things, that the head is responsible for the ethos of the school and the quality of life which goes on there. He is responsible for the curriculum in content, co-ordination, organisation and teaching methods. He is also responsible for the relationships with parents and other adults who are part of the community the school serves. For these reasons therefore it is believed that a decision on school relationships and the curriculum is the headteacher's and, though heads known to us have consulted their staffs and their parents, this still has not taken the ultimate decision away from the head. If the head of a school does not believe that the extension to the curriculum under discussion is in the best interests of the children in his school then he is wise to leave it out and concentrate on those areas of knowledge which he believes his school should impart.

If, however, after due thought and reading, and discussions with colleagues, advisers or inspectors, a head believes that this knowledge could be incorporated into the learning in his school, then he will need to consider the best way to go about this.

The first and obvious point to consider is the attitudes of members of the staff. Just as we believe a head should be free to make decisions on curriculum for his school, so will most heads feel it is desirable to leave the teachers reasonably free to decide on curriculum within the classroom or other unit of organisation for learning. In an area of learning requiring sensitivity and an awareness of its relevance to all learning, the teacher's willingness to include the subject and her attitude to it are vitally important. It seems to us that not only is it professionally wrong to require a teacher to teach any subject which is not in accord with her belief in its relevance for children but, in this case, it could be most undesirable. If the attitudes and values engendered are as important as the facts imparted, then there is little to be gained if a teacher includes the theory but shows little sensitivity to feelings or even worse shows embarrassment or inhibition. It is better left out for the period the children are with such a teacher. At the same time it is an important part of considerate relationships that such a teacher is not allowed to feel a failure or in any way inadequate.

There are schools where excellent work has been done where not all members of staff felt able to participate. In one such school the deputy remained outside the discussions, the decision-making, planning, the parents' meetings and the actual school work with the children and yet so sound were the relationships within the school that he was able to continue to make his contribution to children's learning in other ways.

Although it is not within our own experience, it is possible to envisage a situation where a head may feel that a member of his staff, although willing to include this area of learning in the curriculum, is not the sort of person whom he would wish to work with children in this field. If this should be the case, then a head will need to be firm and organise the learning in the school in such a way that the specific, structured learning is covered by other teachers or the head himself. Incidental learning at infant level or incidental follow-on learning later will always depend on the attitude of a teacher, and a head will need to judge how much a teacher will bring in incidental learning with balance if the subject is part of more planned learning in another part of the school. This is, as one has stated, an uncommon situation which is likely to be most unusual in a school where a head has been fostering sound human relationships.

When, as occasionally happens, a head has a school with a high proportion of older, traditionally-minded teachers who are not open to new ideas then he has either to cover the learning himself, once he has established a close relationship with children, or he must bide his time and delay this extension to the curriculum. When he is able to appoint new staff he can interview bearing this area of the curriculum in mind, with all the others, and the need to appoint staff who show an ability to foster considerate relationships with children.

In one school teachers felt more secure when the head arranged for parents to see the radiovision filmstrips with their own children after school so that the responsibility for follow-up work and answering questions was clearly shared. It is likely that teachers learned much of the children's reactions and of the kind of questions asked from this arrangement and as a result some might well feel able to work with the children in a normal school setting on subsequent occasions. If a head feels that this arrangement, which gives shared responsibility, is the only approach he can make, it seems better to offer children knowledge this way than not at all, but because it is making this learning an occasion, different and special, it will be more difficult to incorporate it into the whole learning incidentally and then in a more organised way, and therefore it seems desirable to avoid this arrangement if possible.

An important factor is the degree of support staff give to this. We have found that a head can very well include this learning in the school curriculum if an adequate number of teachers are willing to participate and those who are unwilling to be personally involved will support the work of others and not go against it in any way. It has, however, been noticed that a number of teachers, who were at first unwilling, changed their minds when they saw colleagues' work and found it to be so interesting to children and not as difficult as they had at first anticipated.

At primary, first and middle school stages of learning it seems most desirable that this topic should be taken by the teacher who normally teaches the class or learning unit so that it is treated in the same way as any other subject. It does not matter whether this is a man or a woman, whether the teacher be married or single, old, young or middle-aged. The important factor is the teacher's relationship with the children and the sort of atmosphere which is engendered day by day. One can think of schools where this learning takes place successfully with teachers of all kinds and ages. In one school it is with a young man with more secondary experience than primary, in others with young women teachers both married and single, in others with older women teachers and teachers near retirement and men who are young, middle-aged or near retirement. Age and sex are of no consequence. Sympathy for and understanding of children are the important factors. For this reason teachers in their first year of teaching may lack confidence to tackle this and will need to be helped by their heads and colleagues.

Some colleges of education have introduced this aspect of the curriculum to students and many have given the whole subject thoughtful consideration. Where students have had ample opportunity to discuss the matter in small groups they seem to have been helped to appreciate the sensitivity and yet candour which this learning requires.

Many head teachers have introduced this topic informally to their staffs and then held discussions with them together or in groups. It has usually been found most helpful to show teachers the visual aids material now available. Our experience has been mostly with the BBC material and we have found that, though the programmes were in the first place made to assist teachers to convey this knowledge to children, it has also helped teachers' own thinking in this field and enabled them to plan for the incorporation of this learning in different ways. It has helped to make a breakthrough in teachers' traditional thinking.

The books in Appendix C should if possible be available on the staff room bookshelf for teachers to read about the subject and its place in education for themselves. They could probably be borrowed if necessary from the local School of Education library. The books in Appendix B will give teachers background knowledge relevant to primary children's interests and suggest approaches and relevant contexts. These books will need to be available to children too.

We are more aware now than in former years of the importance of sound home and school relationships. We appreciate that it is in children's best interest when parents understand the school's aims and know their children's teachers. In this area of knowledge co-operation between parents and teachers is particularly valuable. For this reason it seems wise for heads to inform parents of the work the school is considering undertaking. When parents are informed of the school's approaches to other learning, e.g. mathematics, environmental studies, school journeys and French, etc., this is going to be easier than for schools which do not yet involve parents in their children's school life. There is however evidence from newly appointed heads, who consulted with parents on this topic early on in their first year of appointment, that this promoted mutual regard and parent/teacher co-operation more successfully than they had believed possible.

Letters, notices and invitations from schools to homes are tangible links between the two which can influence relationships more than we have sometimes realised. It has not been uncommon in the past for some schools to send letters home which seemed peremptory to the recipient. Heads who are aware of the importance of teacher/parent co-operation and mutual understanding frame their letters to parents with courtesy, without any loss of clarity and firmness. This letter was sent by the head of a junior mixed and infant school working in old and overcrowded buildings. The letter refers to the subject under discussion. It is simply written so that it can be readily understood by all parents but is without condescension. The school's proposal is definitely stated but the tone of the letter is considerate and courteous.

Dear Parents,

Sex Education in the Primary School

The school has purchased the two educational films 'Growing Up' and 'Where Do Babies Come From?' and we propose to include these in the school curriculum.

I would like you to have the opportunity to see these films for yourselves, and therefore invite you to a preview in the Dining Hall at ——— Road. Due to limited accommodation there will be two showings of these films on the following dates:

Parents of 2nd, 3rd and 4th year Juniors
Friday 27th February at 7.45 p.m.

*Parents of Infants and 1st year Juniors
Friday 6th March at 7.45 p.m.

*These parents are invited to see the films as we wish every parent to have the opportunity. This does not mean that the children in these age groups will necessarily see the films at present.

Mrs. ———, Primary Schools' Adviser, will be present at the meeting on 27th February.

I do hope you will be able to come.

Yours sincerely,

Headmaster.

The tone of invitations and letters of all kinds probably has great influence on the attitude with which parents and teachers come together at meetings. As this is an area where some adults feel very emotional and we all have strong feelings, particular care with letters on this subject seems very worth while.

A good way to help parents to understand a school's approach is to show them the books the children will use and any visual aids material which children see or will see in the course of their learning. The BBC material has not only helped teachers to work with children on this topic, it has also helped parents to understand the approach a school is going to take or is taking. Many parents do not understand what a school is aiming to do in this field. Some are concerned already about the way sex impinges on children in advertising and film display hoardings, etc., and they begin to wonder if schools too are being affected by the current trends. They are invariably reassured by seeing learning material for themselves. In our experience, the reaction of the majority of parents has been one of real pleasure in the material itself and appreciation of the school's sensitive and child-centred approach. Many have said that the material has helped them to understand how to talk to their own children. They find the vocabulary helpful. Further assistance to parents is given in one authority by its School Library Service and the provision in all children's public libraries throughout the county of the books the teachers are likely to use in many schools and which are made available for parents and children. Parents are given a list of those books by the head and it is suggested that they read the book with the child or use the books to find out information with him. A very positive policy of co-operation between parents and teachers is encouraged.

The writer has had experience of meetings with parents in a large number of schools of different kinds: two-form entry urban schools and larger schools, small rural schools, schools receiving children of mostly professional and educated parents and schools receiving children of unskilled workers and manual labourers. Many schools have a mixed intake. There have been common factors in these meetings and two observations can be made.

The first observation is that there exists a most marked correlation between the head's conviction of the rightness of the step he is proposing to take and the willingness of parents to co-operate with him in this. Where a head can explain in simple terms sound educational reasons for an extension of curriculum into this area of personal relationships and answer parents' questions straightforwardly, the great majority of parents are glad to accept the head's ideas. This first observation seems to encourage a policy which gives a head ample opportunity to discuss with colleagues, offers guidance and makes advice available but requires him to think things out in relation to his particular school and come to an independent decision.

There is some evidence which suggests that a head who has not thought this through sufficiently thoroughly and is persuaded by the decision of colleagues or by other influences to talk to parents, and then reveals any uncertainty, creates anxiety in parents. It is worth remembering here that it is contrary to educational practice in this country for a head to call a meeting of parents to assess their views on methods and seek their permission to extend the curriculum. The curriculum is a professional matter and, though a head may be guided by parents' wishes and he may indeed invite them to express their views in order to assess their support, he nevertheless is expected by parents, and quite rightly, to be able to offer them professional guidance and give them information. They do not expect to be asked to express views on what a head should allow to be taught and to put them in such a position strains their confidence in a school.

The second observation is that parents tend on the whole to ask the same questions. The most common question or comment concerns the radiovision programme 'Where Do Babies Come From?'. This shows a concern for the fact that the commentary excludes any reference to falling in love, of love between parents or that intercourse is a part of a deeply loving relationship. It is necessary for a head to be able to explain that the material is designed to meet the emotional and intellectual needs of children of about seven to ten years of age for whom the experience of love is that which is received from parents, and perhaps grandparents and others. In his own way the head will help parents to realise that, on the whole, children's experience of love is that of warm feelings engendered by different intimate occasions such as bedtime, returning home after an absence, the receipt of gifts and birthday presents, of fun and larky horseplay with father—all different ways of receiving love and thereby learning to give love. When a head can help parents to understand that sexual love between adults is not within the compass of children's experience, although they have rudimentary sexual feelings, we have found that the large majority of parents, in fact all but one or two in an occasional meeting, are able to understand the sound reasons why love is not explicitly stated but strongly implied. Often parents see this clearly when one can convey the idea that we, as adults, probably want to include this as a kind of insurance, something we feel we should state to make us feel we have done our duty— put ourselves in the clear, so to speak. This can be part of an attitude summed up by 'Well, I did tell him/her so it is not my fault'. When parents are able to view the 'Merry-Go-Round' programmes on 16mm film they are assured that at this stage family life is repeatedly portrayed.

This is often followed by questions on how the morality of human sexual behaviour is to be conveyed. An explanation of how aesthetic and moral understanding is developed in the adolescent and post-adolescent years assists parents to understand how the school aligns its teaching with the children's normal development and their first-hand experience of a loving home and similar influences and why there are few rules and precepts stated but family feelings strongly implied. Sometimes it helps to bear in mind that the 1964 Government Survey among parents of primary school children reports 8 per cent of families as being without one or both natural parents. This can be three or four children in some classes. Also some immigrant children come from families whose marriage customs are different from our own.

The maturity of the head and the parents' trust in his or her judgment in all things related to their children will obviously influence their attitude.

Parents then nearly always want to know when the head is going to include this learning in the school curriculum and at what ages he proposes to offer children specific theoretical information. Sometimes they want to know the context in which information will be given and how children will be prepared to receive it.

It is noticeable that parents do not usually want to be given a detailed outline of a scheme of work but assurances that this learning will be given in a sensitive and appropriate way which seems relevant to their children. Some parents have said that they would like to talk about the subject first so that they themselves have partly prepared their child to receive structured, planned information in school. Other parents have said that they have always answered their children's questions when asked. Many are reassured when a head can tell them that he believes that this is a very good thing and that close co-operation between parents and teachers is particularly valuable in this learning and that what is best for the child is when a school builds on the foundations laid in a good home. Many parents are glad to accept this partnership and be assured that the school is not opposing, ignoring or taking over the parents' responsibilities but supporting them. Other parents are in a sense grateful that the school, with its particular understanding of children, is going to introduce their child to a subject which they have found difficulty in broaching.

The majority of parents have accepted the head's suggestions on the approximate ages when children will be introduced to specific theory. It has not been unusual however for a few, usually more educated parents, to suggest that an introduction to the story of where babies come from should be made at an earlier stage than the head is suggesting as they believe that an open and frank approach from the earliest years is desirable.

Although more and more schools now have different programmes to familiarise parents with school practice and organisation, etc., there are still many parents who come into their child's school with adverse feelings. Such feelings are caused by memories of their own school experiences under more authoritarian régimes than we would sanction now. From their own experience of school they have a somewhat vague idea that their children are going to be instructed in a rather formal way, that spellings will be drilled and the facts tested. They envisage the child being made anxious if he does not understand everything immediately and answer up readily. One has found that a short clear statement on contemporary practice is reassuring and that parents' attitudes change quite markedly when they are told that the story of babies is offered to children to accept or reject in the same way as any other story, poem or piece of music or other similar experience is. They are relieved to be told categorically that this learning is offered and not forced, that testing is inappropriate and that a child is free to use it to grow on in whatever way suits his own individuality. Sometimes a clear statement on lines similar to this helps parents to realise that they do not have to protect their children in any way and that indeed the school is as concerned for their children's welfare as they are.

Two questions which sometimes arise need careful consideration. The first is a question from parents who have an adopted child and want to know how they can answer their child's questions. In helping adoptive parents with this problem it seems wise to consider these points. Firstly, the theory is truthful and true of all people born into the world and therefore true for the adopted child. Secondly, the adopted child is different in one way only and a rather special way and that is that he has been chosen by a mother to be her own because the mother in whose uterus he grew could not keep him. The child's well-being, happiness and acceptance of this fact is dependent on his belief in his value to his adopted mother and father. An adopted child, for a while, may deliberately seek assurance of his adoptive parents' love and be helped to accept his own circumstances by perhaps a more overt expression of love than the legitimate child needs because he takes it for granted.

It is important to understand that the adopted child needs to know the truth about himself but also needs to believe that he is valued and loved so that when he accepts the truth he does not feel rejected.

The second question which requires careful consideration is similar and comes from foster-parents. Here again one needs to be certain that it is understood that one must be truthful and that the story of where babies come from is true for us all. The foster-parents' position is in many ways more difficult than that of adoptive parents, for though circumstances differ, in most cases they show their love for their foster-child but at the same time they have to control any possessive feelings they may have for the child and help him to preserve a memory of his real mother to whom he could be returned. They have to help him to accept that he has two mothers, a natural mother and a foster-mother.

Perhaps his possession of two mothers can be a sort of compensation to a child though it probably should not be overstressed. What one must face here is that all children want to know how they came into the world and be assured that their birth was like the births of all babies, and adopted and foster-children need this information as much as other children. They do have to come to terms with a fact that their own mother could not keep them and this means the acceptance of being rejected or partly rejected. This is faced at different stages in development according to the personality and circumstances of the individual but the ability to cope with this situation and accept it is certainly dependent on an adequate self-image, a belief that one is valued, and this will be given to the child by the attitude of his adoptive parents or foster-parents and others whom he values and loves. A child who grows up into the truth about himself so that he gradually comes to terms with his own situation will not be vulnerable to the dangerously traumatic experience of the child who suddenly learns of his adopted status by accident. Also in many ways it is easier for us all to show warmth and love through feelings and physical contact to young children. The hugs and cuddles come with spontaneity and are usually received in similar spirit. The child builds up a sense of his own worth from these experiences in early years which is likely to see him through adolescence when the overt gestures of love from the family are usually less acceptable.

It has seemed to us that there is a very marked change in parents' thinking and attitudes now compared with a few years ago. We have found that there has been parental opposition from only an occasional individual parent or couple who seem to have made a personal adjustment to life which precludes the ability to reconsider attitudes or think about how such attitudes were developed. Such individuals nearly always retain these attitudes for emotional reasons, often from experience in early years of life and as a result their reactions are emotional. It will be noticed that often such an individual or couple will raise objections early on in a meeting because they feel so emotional about it, whereas the less emotional and more thoughtful will be thinking the matter out and will arrive at questions and comments later. A head is wise therefore not to be 'thrown' by an emotional reaction early in a meeting, but to answer questions as clearly as he can and maintain an atmosphere of calm and reason. In our experience such a parent

who has difficulty in accepting new ideas on this subject is then
often helped as much by the comments of other parents who
reveal views contrary to theirs, as by the head of the school. Where
an individual is taking over more than a fair share of discussion
time it seems wise to offer such an individual an appointment to
talk over a personal viewpoint privately. In our experience it is
best to let a meeting continue for as long as parents want to talk,
ask questions or make comments, for this is the best way of sharing
with them the ideas and aims the school has for their children and
once they understand these and there is common ground, mutual
trust and co-operation can develop.

A head will also probably believe it to be in the child's best
interest if he also asks parents who wish to withdraw their child
from this learning to see him personally. In a quiet interview,
sometimes it is a long one, he has the best chance of helping
parents to understand reasons for this inclusion in education and
how impossible it is to keep a child ignorant and how hurtful
it can be to make a primary age child feel different from his
contemporaries. It seems to us desirable, both for the individual
child and for sound educational principles, that a head should do
all that is possible to avoid a child being excluded.

This exclusion is often best avoided by the head showing that
children are curious and want to know and that no head, teacher
or anyone can guarantee to keep a child ignorant. One can go so
far as to say that any child who is kept at home while this learning
is taking place is likely to be the very child who will return to
school and go around to the others with 'Tell me, tell me'. Certainly at some later stage the request will be repeated but, as in
the past, he may have to have recourse to a place behind the
bicycle sheds and receive less accurate and often harmful information without the chance to incorporate these values we
believe should be associated with such knowledge.

Another factor here is that experience shows that this area
of learning is soon incorporated into the general overall learning of children and becomes part of many relevant topics. It
becomes a subject which is discussed by children when they
find it appropriate. This is as it should be. We do not want to
treat this differently from other learning. We do not want to
make it special. Where this learning therefore is most successful
it is likely to be impossible to timetable and hence impossible
to advise parents in advance of a piece of work or topic in order

for them to plan to keep a child away from school.

We have found that parents' attendance at meetings on this area of the curriculum have been much higher than usual, but as is to be expected, few schools have had one hundred per cent of parents present. Provided all parents concerned with the subject have received an invitation to attend and adequate notice has been given, it seems reasonable for a head to assume that he has in the audience those who are concerned and interested and that he must, if he wishes, be guided by their response and not be over concerned by those who are not present. This is not to say that a head should not offer to see parents individually by appointment or make alternative arrangements if he finds that there was another meeting or occasion competing for parents' attention. But it does mean that he should be realistic and not necessarily expect a full attendance to discuss this subject when we do not expect it for others.

There are still some parents who do not feel comfortable in schools and avoid attendance at meetings on any subject. There are large numbers in some areas who trust the head and his staff to know what is best for their children in school hours and do not understand that their views are being sought. There are others who attend meetings more to receive guidance on their children's welfare from heads and teachers than to voice their own views. Heads in these circumstances will need to come to a professional decision and give a tactful but positive lead to parents' thinking in this field as they probably do in other circumstances. Perhaps this headmaster's account is helpful here.

> My school is very much a neighbourhood school on the edge of a smallish country town. By virtue of the rapid development of AERE estates the town was socially polarised. This meant that this school served an estate solely composed of council houses, which has only recently changed as some new private estates have been built.
>
> At this time the best guess would be that the population is 80 per cent—85 per cent class iii and iv, and 15 per cent—20 per cent class ii. In the light of the Newsom reports this is significant since 'working class' attitudes to sex education are more conservative than those of the middle class.
>
> Seen in this setting, the school policy on sex education has two main points. It was thought desirable not only to get the

125

parents' consent but also to involve them actively, and secondly not to overstress sex education but to treat it incidentally, naturally and without embarrassment.

The idea of introducing sex education was discussed in the first instance at staff meetings. Predictably it provoked sharp feelings. While most were agreed that it was desirable, there was considerable doubt about whether it was not really the parents' job, and whether we were in fact doing the parents a disservice by taking over yet another parental duty. A few staff doubted their own ability to take the lessons.

The two radiovision filmstrips, 'Growing Up' and 'Where Do Babies Come From?' were shown to the managers and to a pilot group of parents at a PTA meeting. Both parties fully approved and so a general parents' meeting was called.

At this the parents were shown the filmstrip, and then asked to discuss it. The main points centred on the age at which the films should be shown, the order of the films, the fact that the films had no moral element and scarcely mentioned the importance of marriage and finally whether children were ready for the films at this age (eight years—eleven years). At the end of the meeting, of perhaps 200 parents, only one parent was against showing the films though some were only lukewarm. A second meeting was held so that more parents could see the filmstrips and again about 150 parents attended this.

At these meetings it was stressed that the parents had an important role, and that one of the important functions of these filmstrips was to introduce the subject so that parents could discuss it. The films were designed to give them a 'lead in'.

Accordingly, whenever the films are shown and they are seen by the second, third and fourth years the parents are informed by letter of the day when they will be shown so that they can prepare children for the films if they wish and discuss the films on the day as well.

At the same time about 20—30 books recommended on this subject were introduced into the team libraries. They are freely available for use at any time. The consensus of staff opinion was that the subject should be treated factually, honestly but without emphasis, that in fact both emphasis and evasion were out.

Thus, when children write books about the human body, reproduction is treated as part of it, and equally pets (we have rabbits, guinea-pigs, birds and fish) give rise to queries on sex differences, menstrual flow, twins, differences in gestation periods, and these are answered as they are asked. In literature, 'difficult' biblical passages are not avoided, any more than discussion references to homosexuality and prostitution are ignored.

All members of staff share this attitude. Occasionally newcomers are wary but so far have accepted this easily.

The children seem to have accepted this. I was considerably encouraged by one ten-year-old who came to tell me without any difficulty that Joey had got his penis stuck in the zip on his trousers.

While some of the children show a little embarrassment when they see the films, most of this seems to be because they can see people naked. This happens only in the second year classes. Most of these children, and all the third and fourth years, accept the filmstrips very easily.

Schools are different from each other. Each school is unique. There is no one way of fostering good parent/teacher relationships. Each head will do this in his own way and from his own personality and educational convictions. Research and experience clearly show us that parents who are helped to understand the aims of their child's school and who become involved in their child's education are the parents who are able to be most educationally supporting, with the result that their child is more likely to develop his educational potential.

This field of sex education for young children or, as is more appropriate for these years, knowledge of human beings, babies, 'the story of me', is an area of education where the desirability of partnership between parents and teachers is clearer than in some others. Certainly it is an aspect of knowledge which is being considered more thoroughly and widely now than before and at a time when home and school relationships are being widely considered too. We have found close links between them. Where mutual trust and understanding exist between school and home, parents attend meetings on this part of the curriculum disposed to try to understand because goodwill and trust are already established. Where this topic has been one of the subjects of an early meeting between a new head and parents, and the head has been able to convey sound reasons for wishing to extend the curriculum, this has often engendered mutual regard and trust and got sound relationships off to a good start. In schools with an established pattern of meetings and co-operation, the proposal to extend curriculum has often been a rewarding occasion, for it has revealed parents' trust in head and staff and support for all the school undertakes.

Above all these considerations is the one that the child is likely to grow up with accurate knowledge and an awareness of the values and attitudes most of us would wish to associate with human sexuality when parents and teachers are both concerned with him as an individual. For the child's sake, therefore, it seems to us wise that heads and staffs should explain the school's learning to parents and offer positive suggestions on how one can help the other by doing all they can in their own particular circumstances to bring homes and schools, parents and teachers together.

For the present, however, there will be a few heads in certain areas who will feel that their parents are not yet ready to discuss education in so personal a matter. Such heads will have to decide *in loco parentis*, from a consideration of what seems best for children while in their school. If we believe that all children need this information at appropriate times in their primary and middle school years then indeed children living in crowded and other less favoured conditions probably need accurate knowledge and a place to seek it quite urgently. In these circumstances it seems even more desirable that heads should have opportunities to consult with colleagues, discuss with advisers or inspectors and be supported in their curriculum aims by their education authority so that they are able to feel confident in making a decision to extend the curriculum even when they do not have the clear support of the majority of parents which heads of schools in more favoured areas invariably receive.

Chapter 8

Beyond the primary/middle school

'One of our problems is to derive our ethical and moral thinking and acting from a basic foundation which is a comprehensive view of what we are as human beings and what we want for ourselves and our relationships. I think our concern must rest in a consideration of the quality of relationships which we are able to develop in our families, in our communities, and ultimately, at the international level. When a decision is to be made concerning behaviour I think the moral decision will be confidence and integrity in relationships.'

Dr. L. Kirkendall

The general aim of sex education in the schools described here has been to 'open the door' on to an aspect of the real world which hitherto we have tended to shut out of the primary/middle schools. The inclusion of this aspect of reality into general learning has allowed knowledge to be acquired gradually, when opportune, in the same way as it is acquired about any other aspect of real life. Its place in contexts which are relevant to children's interests,

129

in incidental, then more formal, structured ways has allowed the child to construct an accurate framework of knowledge to which additional theory can be added as the ability to understand complexities develops.

The learning which is appropriate to the majority of children in the primary/middle school is largely concerned with the development of perceptual, practical and simple theoretical concepts. It is important that we recognise that this is only the beginning and that the acquisition of more detailed theory and the development of aesthetic and moral concepts belong to the secondary level of education and beyond, throughout life.

At secondary and higher levels of education we are becoming more aware that, in addition to provision for sound academic learning and intellectual development, we must also find ways of educating young people for contemporary life by incorporating learning which is able to contribute to emotional development. This means among other things, that we need to help young people in their search for identity, to assist them in coming to terms with their own personalities and help them to learn to interact symbiotically with others. We also need to support them in their development of personal ideals and a code of behaviour relevant to daily life.

Some young people in secondary schools, colleges and later in adult life will develop aesthetic and moral concepts of complexity and sophistication. Others may develop such concepts in simple terms only and will need positive guidance and help if they are to relate aesthetic and moral ideas in a practical way to themselves and apprehend their relevance to their own lives.

With our traditional academically-based teaching in literature and drama in particular, and in music, the arts and languages, the most able have always been exposed to influences which have contributed to their personal development. Because the less academically gifted have not been able to profit by studies of this complexity, they have not been exposed to the same subtle cultural and moral influences. We realise more clearly now than in earlier years that it is important to find approaches which will bring more young people to an awareness of these influences and give them a better chance of developing wider facets of personality and maturity. At the same time perhaps we are wise to bear in mind that part of learning in these fields is through feeling as well as reasoning and that this is true for all levels of intellectual ability. To foster intellectual growth and ignore personal emotional facets in the most able has not always been conducive to their full development and maturity.

Personal and emotional needs and fostering an awareness of the importance of human relationships are less likely to be met in class-based learning situations than in discussion groups with an understanding adult. A few secondary schools now have counsellors who work in the field of human relationships. Others value the help of tutors of the National Marriage Guidance Council who, with their training for this work, are often ideally suited to working with young people who want to be assured of confidentiality. More and more schools are becoming aware that, within the traditionally accepted field of pastoral care, ways must be found of helping teachers to work more informally with young people and on a more reciprocal basis than hitherto. These teachers will need to have sympathy for and understanding of young people and the skill to develop relationships which will enable them to show an understanding of the particular problems of personal development. In addition they will need the ability to identify the general problems of young people growing up in a rapidly changing society and be able to help them to come to terms with them. Pupils in school today are going to become part of a society where the adults themselves find it difficult to ascertain the future, what occupations men and women of the coming generation will fill, what relationships they will have with each other, what effect easily available contraception will have on the role of nearly all women, and what view society will take of marriage. Our view of marriage is certainly changing but it doesn't appear to be undermined by change. On the contrary, it appears to be more highly regarded than ever. Given more opportunities to acquire understanding of ourselves and others, it could be that this still most permanent and personal of all relationships, a love between two people which is capable of modification and development throughout life from young adulthood through to middle age and old age, will remain an ideal to which many more will aspire. Such a relationship seems to be still best described by Paul to the Corinthians in this modern version:

> Love is patient and kind, love is not jealous, or conceited or proud, love is not ill-mannered, or selfish, or irritable, love does not keep a record of wrongs, love is not happy with

evil, but is happy with truth. Love never gives up: its faith, hope and patience never fail.

In a more contemporary setting it is interesting to note that in 1966, in Education Pamphlet No. 49, Health in Education, it is suggested that Margaret Mead and other anthropologists have defined these demanding interdependent roles for men and women today which most of us are likely to recognise as still true:

> A woman needs lover, tender friend, supporter, defender, big boy in need of occasional comforting, constant companion, father of her children and herself. The man looks for mistress, beloved companion, adviser and comforter, frail clinging protégée, playmate and mother of his children and himself.

Certainly we can see that adolescents now in our schools will need, as adults, to be able to make rational decisions on matters which radically affect their lives and the lives of others which their parents were not called upon to make with such urgency. For instance, for sound demographic reasons, as well as personal ones, young people will need to decide on the number of children they will have. They will be helped to do this if they know the facts such as the country's and world birth-rates, death-rates, food production and other relevant statistics. To come to an intelligent decision on the contraceptive pill needs scientific knowledge, a concept of probability and understanding of relative risks.

Rational decisions can only be made with knowledge. Secondary schools must provide the means for pupils to acquire this knowledge so that rational decision-making, relevant to the present day, becomes possible for as many as possible. Many of the guides and outlines for work in Nuffield Secondary Science and the General Studies Project and Humanities Project of the Schools' Council include approaches to themes which the discerning teacher could engineer to encourage development of these abilities.

Moral decision-making, too, which is made on rational grounds is more likely to be a firm guide for life without being inappropriately inflexible than decision-making under duress, feelings of guilt, fear and retribution. Many teachers are likely to find the material from the Schools' Council's Moral Education Project helpful, while some may find fresh insight from accounts of the work of the Farmington Trust on Moral Education. The Schools' Broadcasting Council of the BBC and Independent Television Authority offer valuable aids to teachers to help them to stimulate group discussion on contemporary personal problems and human relationships. This is particularly helpful in relation to the raising of the school leaving age. Programmes are on television and BBC radio.

In all the changes through which we are passing there does seem to be emerging a fairly common factor in our moral code. We seem to be moving towards becoming a more caring society and to appreciate the importance of considerate relationships for full development of individuals and for the well-being of groups of all kinds.

The quality of human relationships derived from values which enable us to give care, consideration and concern for others are the most important ingredients of education in life and for life, and must include understanding of human sexuality. With the growing awareness of this it becomes clear that this subject cannot be defined as a body of knowledge only, even though it is indeed a science with a precise terminology. It is much more than this in also being a fundamental and deep emotional experience for which fulfilment is not dependent on accurate scientific knowledge though to have a degree of such knowledge is probably desirable. As educationalists we shall need to be able to convey that sexual fulfilment is much more dependent on an understanding and acceptance of oneself as an individual, an appreciation of the feelings and aspirations of one's fellows, the willingness to give generously before one can receive, tolerance and an awareness of the common bond of humanity.

We shall need to be aware of the many other facets of human sexuality including those which assist our own creative impulses as well as being the inspiration for artists of all kinds. We shall need to appreciate that sex is simple, basic and common in being part of the fabric of daily life and yet it is at the same time inextricably part of human aspiration, imagination, inspiration and religious belief. All these and others are most complex concepts to which we are ever adding new dimensions.

The responsibility for opening up avenues for discovery, exploration and understanding of these complexities lies with secondary and further education and may be part of many subjects and disciplines. It is becoming clearer that part of our success may be related to how well we are able to convey that our sexuality is a part of our personal development all our lives; to be influenced by painting, sculpture, music, drama, literature, architecture and all those features in nature which move us or which we find beautiful. And lastly, in addition to this, for most of us, the most potent influence of all lies in the quality of our own relationships with all whose lives impinge upon our own and our ability to sustain them by our own integrity.

Appendices

Appendix A

Books for young children

It is suggested that those marked with * should be given priority in selecting for purchase for class libraries. Parents often like to know about these books either to purchase or to borrow from public libraries.

The Wonderful Story of How You Were Born, S. M. Gruenberg (World's Work).
One of the best books for children to read for themselves. Written with real understanding of young children's development.

How a Baby is Born, K. de Schweinitz (Routledge & Kegan Paul).
One of the earlier books. Very good for class, group and individual use in the junior school. 'This book tells how we became alive, and are born and grow up.'

Biology, Ames and Wyler (Hamlyn).
A large attractive book for both browsing and obtaining information.

Peter and Caroline, Sten Hegeler (Tavistock).
A good story book for infants which the teacher could read to the children in groups and they could later read themselves.

Affords an opportunity for the teacher to show her willingness to answer children's questions, discuss personal relationships and help the child towards a development of sound attitudes. From such an introduction information on human life and reproduction could continue to be given according to interest and stages of development. A good book to recommend to parents.

How the Baby Came, Dorotheen Allan and Marie Neurath (Heinemann).
A family story of Mummy, Daddy, John and Mary and how their new baby brother was born. Well written and clearly illustrated. Reads aloud well for infants and is a good class library book for lower juniors.

Like *Peter and Caroline*, the story gives the teacher an opportunity to introduce the subject and show her willingness to discuss personal interests with the children if they wish.

How John Grew an Inch, D. Allan and M. Neurath (Heinemann).
Similar to the previous one, concentrating on growing.

Dan Berry's New Baby, Anthony Jones (Blackie).
One of four supplementary readers in a series on real life situations, 'Life with Dan Berry'. Suitable for reading to younger children and for children of about eight years to read to themselves. All four books could be in the class library.

How Babies are Made, A. Andry and S. Schepp (Time-Life International).
A fairly good book for parents to read with children from about the age of three, for teachers to use with groups of infants and for children to use themselves throughout the primary school. A very simple account which answers the main questions children are known to ask, written with advice from the Child Study Association of America. Illustrations are in paper sculpture and on the whole illustrate the text well.

The Birth of Sunset's Kittens, Carla Stevens. Photographs, Leonard Stevens (World's Work).
A delightful book for infants and lower juniors. A detailed sequence of photgraphs and a simple short text describing the birth of kittens to Sunset, the tabby cat. The likeness to human birth is explicitly stated. The account is warm and child-centred. Excellent for quiet reading with groups followed by discussion.

How You Began, Hilary Spiers (Dent).
Simple outline for pre-school children and infants in school. A good book to recommend to parents to read with children at home and for a teacher to use in recapitulating on this early learning or to introduce these ideas with children in a school setting. To an adult some illustrations seem crude in colour and drawing.

Where Do Babies Come From? Margaret Sheffield (Jonathan Cape).
A first-class story-book of the BBC filmstrip and therefore invaluable for use with it in both homes and schools.

Appendix B

Books for junior/middle school children

Peter and Pamela Grow Up, H. W. Tame (Darwen Finlayson).
Written for eleven-year-olds by a primary school headmaster as a basis for his own school's course on reproduction and for children to read for themselves to recapitulate and ponder. The introduction is sound and helpful for heads and teachers. The text and diagrams convey with accuracy and simplicity just the right amount of information for the majority of primary school children to understand. This knowledge will form a firm basis for information of greater detail at the secondary stage.

This is the result of five years' experience and is an excellent book for the teacher and for the class library.

Time to Grow Up, H. W. Tame (Macmillan).
Written by a primary school headmaster and Marriage Guidance Counsellor for junior school children. A clear factual account of growth and sexual development with explicit reference to human emotions and behaviour in contemporary society. The self-control necessary for our protracted education for adult life is stressed, and adults' responsibility for babies and young children over many years is explicitly stated. The book keeps to its main theme

of human development. An excellent class library book and one to recommend to parents for reading and discussion in the home.

The Human Body, Cyril Bibby and Ian T. Morison (Puffin).
Good, clear diagrams. Excellently balanced material. Simple but accurate. Clear presentation of vocabulary. Excellent value. Sound source book for teachers. Good class library book for juniors. Good introduction to group discussion which could develop into class or group lesson. Sound recapitulation for the individual child.

Right from the Start, E. R. Matthews (Barrie and Rockliff).
A very good handbook for the teacher and a good book for the junior class library. Clearly told and well balanced. Human reproduction is described in the context of evolution and animal life. A detailed account, simply written, of conception, pregnancy and birth. Adequate black-and-white diagrams and photographs. Good value.

Your Body, A Ladybird Book, Series 536 (Wills and Hepworth).
**Where Do Babies Come From?* Jill Kenner (NMGC).
The author is a Marriage Guidance Education Counsellor and it is from her experience of discussion work in personal relationships with young people and the questions children have asked her that this booklet has been written. It is designed for nine- to twelve-years-olds and incorporates answers to the questions primary school children so often ask.
A booklet to recommend to parents.

Growing Up, I. Arneil, B. Marshall and W. Marshall (Nelson).
Health Education for Schools Books I and II, Books III and IV. Attractively presented, easy to read books for junior school children which present an introduction to health education in the broad context of everyday life situations and human relationships. Useful book to suggest to teachers, starting points for discussion and discovery and for children to have in the class library. These books make a positive contribution towards the development of personal identity.

Programmed Sex Information (Longman).
A graded series of booklets designed to answer the simple questions presented on where babies come from, birth, growth and adolescence. The text consists of question and answer and clear diagrammatic illustrations and contemporary photographs. The

aim is to present factual information alone. The books would be very useful in a class library to assist recapitulation of facts which have already been conveyed in a context of care and concern but some of the other children's books which set the information in a more 'feeling context' should also be available.

i) *Babies and Families*, Anne Kind and John Leedham.
Human and animal babies, human and animal adults. Male and female lions and a lion family. Human male and female. Parents and families.

(ii) *You Begin Life*, Dr. R. Kind and J. Leedham.
A new-born baby. Baby growing in the uterus. Very clear diagrams of birth of a baby.

iii) *You Grow Up*, Dr. R. Kind and J. Leedham.
Physical development in puberty with clear diagrams. Menstruation. Differences between male and female. Clear statement of intercourse in simple sentences and a magnified picture of fertilisation.

These books are probably best suited to ten- and eleven-year-olds as a means of recapitulating previous learning. Books 4 and 5 are for secondary age pupils.

How You Are Made, Hilary Spiers (Dent) (adaptation of a book by C. Palmgreen).
Describes in straightforward rather conversational language information on human anatomy and systems, including excretory and reproductive. The style and content are geared to children between eight and twelve years and prepare the way for more common biological terminology later. It is a matter-of-fact book for junior children. Adults used only to conventional biology text books will find the language chatty.

The First Cry, Colette Pontal (Dent).
The writer is also the illustrator. It is a personal account of the development of a human being from conception to birth. It deserves a place in all primary school libraries for its sensitive awareness of young children's interest in the baby *in utero*. Correct terminology is admirably used. The text will be fully comprehended by average ten- and eleven-year-olds, but younger children will also choose the book and grow with it, reading more each time. It conveys care for the young without sentimentality and will be a valuable addition to children's books which appropriately convey feelings and facts together.

Appendix C

Books for adults

The following books give in simple terms the kind of information primary school children want to know.

The Wonder of Life, Milton I. Levine and Jean H. Seligman (Routledge and Kegan Paul).
How we are born and how we grow up. Clearly written and helpful book for teachers with little knowledge of the subject. The approach is excellent for nine- to twelve-year-olds and within the text answers questions which often confuse young people. It will give teachers the detailed background necessary to meet the interests and answer the questions which arise when this learning is introduced. The vocabulary is appropriate without unnecessary medical terms. There is a helpful glossary. The book could well be made available to the children although only the most able will be able to use it on their own.

Right from the Start, E. R. Matthews (Barrie and Rockliff).
See p. 142

The Human Body, Cyril Bibby and Ian T. Morison (Puffin).
See p. 142

How a Baby is Born, K. de Schweinitz (Routledge and Kegan Paul).
See p. 137

The Wonderful Story of How You Were Born, S. M. Gruenberg (World's Work).
See p. 137
Very useful for teachers to read for the insight it gives into a sound approach rather than for factual information.

Peter and Pamela Grow Up, H. W. Tame (Darwen Finlayson).
See p. 141

Time to Grow Up, H. W. Tame (Macmillan).
See p. 141

Sex Education, Cyril Bibby (Macmillan).
One of the earlier textbooks for teachers now in its 8th edition. Covers sex education in secondary schools more fully than in primary but is nevertheless a helpful book for primary teachers. The emphasis on personal relationships is much less than in more recent books on the subject but it may provide a link for young teachers between the sex education they received themselves and the subject in the context of personal relationships as we are considering it today. For this reason it could be helpful in formulating principles to guide us in the work with young children. *For teachers only, not for children's use.*

Animal Babies, Alice Day Pratt. New edition (Darwen Finlayson).
The Family Finds Out, Edith Fisher Hunter; *Always Growing*, Elizabeth M. Manwell, both Beacon Press, Boston, U.S.A.
Martin and Judy, Vol. I 3–4, Verna Hills Bayley; Vol. II 4–5, Verna Hills Bayley; Vol. III 5–6, Verna Hills Bayley; all Beacon Press, Boston, U.S.A.
The six books set out to meet the needs and to allay the anxieties of young children, which arise in the family and later in school in making personal relationships with adults, siblings, new babies and animals and in understanding life and living in all its aspects. The birth of young animals, the death of a pet, the preparation for and the birth of a new baby are included in the family-centred stories. They are exceedingly valuable as examples of a way in which children can be helped to make relationships and acquire attitudes of concern for others and consideration. They have an ethical purpose.

They provide the kind of setting in infant classes in which children's questions can be answered and, more important still, offer the child the opportunity to ask his own questions which he may have suppressed because of adult inhibition or lack of awareness of this need. By the use of these types of stories a parent and/or teacher is able to show the child their willingness to give information on deeply felt aspects of living, including human reproduction, but at the same time a balance is preserved so that the information given can be relevant to the child's needs.

The stories are written for American children and the vernacular is unsuitable for children in this country. Infant teachers will, however, find them helpful and language will be easily modified by a good story teller. They can be obtained on loan from many Education Libraries.

Appendix D

Background reading for teachers

A Textbook of Sex Education, Julia Dawkins (Blackwell).
A very good book for teachers. Sex education is clearly shown to be the understanding of factual information in the context of an awareness of human qualities of care and concern for others. Teachers are given guidance in approaching this part of the curriculum with sensitivity and the appropriate approach at various stages of development from pre-school child to adolescence.

Love and Sex in Plain Language, Eric Johnson (André Deutsch).
This is all the title suggests. It is written for secondary school children in a simple straightforward way to prepare them for the physical and emotional changes ahead. It is a useful book for primary school teachers as an excellent example of a way of conveying factual information with understanding for personal feelings.

Sex Education and the New Morality (Columbia University Press).
A search for a meaningful social ethic. Child Study Association of America.

Accounts by five participants of a conference held by the Association expressing views from the fields of psychiatry, social work, education and religious education.

'One of our problems is to derive our ethical and moral thinking and acting from a basic foundation which is a comprehensive view of what we are as human beings, and what we want out of ourselves and our relationships. I think our concern must rest in a consideration for the quality of relationships which we are able to develop in our families, in our communities, and ultimately, at the international level. When a decision is to be made concerning behaviour I think the moral decision will be the one which works towards the creation of trust, confidence and integrity in relationships.' Dr. L. Kirkdendall, Professor of Family Life, Oregon State University.

What to tell your Children about Sex (Allen and Unwin). Child Study Association of America.

A most valuable book for teachers and for recommendation to parents. This is an outline of emotional and intellectual development with special reference to the child's own sexual development, his sexual interests and the questions he will need answered at the various stages of his growth. The human qualities of love, tender regard and sex as an expression of the desire to find meaning and worth in another person are implicit throughout.

'The book covers the various stages of personality development from infancy through adolescence. It tries to weave sex, as an aspect of love, into this pattern of growth.'

Though written for American parents and teachers it is of equal value to us.

The Sexual Behaviour of Young People, Michael Schofield (Longman and Penguin).

An account of the research by the Health Education Council supported by the Nuffield Foundation. The research covered more than 1,800 boys and girls and elicited the facts about the source of their knowledge of sexual matters, the education they had received and their attitudes. It has revealed the defects in educational provision in this area and has influenced rethinking at secondary and primary level. A book which all teachers should read for sound background information.

Towards a Quaker View of Sex, Friends House, Euston Road, London, NW1. Revised edition 1964.

An essay by a group of Friends.

'Those who read this essay with care will realise that we are asking for an approach that starts from something deeper than a conventional moral judgment: rather it is from a concern for full responsibility in personal relationship.'

'The essay does not pretend to be a set of ultimate conclusions; it invites the help of those who read it in carrying forward the exercise of thought and prayer in which the authors have engaged.' Preface to second edition.

Sex Education in Schools, Church Information Office, Church House, Westminster, SW1.

Sex Education in Primary School, Albert G. Chanter (Macmillan, 1966).

A fairly recent account of a primary school headmaster's experience of giving specific instruction in sex education in his junior mixed school. Practical, helpful and contemporary. Shows the muddle and confusion of young children and perhaps, therefore, implies sound reasons why schools should help in this aspect of learning.

The Individual, Sex and Society, edited by C. B. Broderick and J. Barnard (Johns Hopkins Press).

A handbook for teachers and counsellors produced by SIECUS, the Sex Information and Education Council for the United States, in response to the need for a more extensive and reliable body of information for teachers. It is intended for a textbook for training teachers to teach mainly older children in US maintained schools. Nevertheless teachers in this country may find some of the ideas and much of the information helpful. It is obtainable from many School of Education Libraries.

Teachers as Counsellors, Alick Holden (Constable).

Understanding Sex: A Young Person's Guide, Alan F. Guttmacher (Allen & Unwin).

Personal Values in the Modern World, M. V. C. Jeffreys (Penguin).

Sex in Society, Alex Comfort (Duckworth).

Health in Education, Education Pamphlet No. 49 (HMSO).

Sex and Society, Dr. Helena Wright (Allen and Unwin).

Introduction to Moral Education, Wilson, Williams, Sugarman (Penguin).

Keeping Animals in Schools.
A handbook for teachers published by the Department of Education and Science.

Sex Education in Perspective 1972 (NMGC).
A symposium on work in progress.

Appendix E

Three programmes

Programme S9A

1. Read the information in Column A.
2. Complete the sentence in Column B by choosing a word or number from Column C.
3. **Write out the whole sentence for your notes—do not write on this programme.**
4. Check answers from Check list.
5. Do post-test. (Do not write on the post-test paper.)
6. Check answers to post-test.

The Reproductive System

A	B	C
Read this	**Complete this**	**Choose one of these to complete B**
1. All living creatures reproduce themselves.	All l***** creatures reproduce themselves.	Lazy Living Human
2. **Reproduction** means the handing on of life.	The handing on of l*** is called Reproduction.	Life Food Sex
3. The handing on of life is called **Reproduction.**	Re********** is the handing on of life.	Reproduction Digestion Sex

153

4. Some of the lower forms of life (e.g. Amoeba) reproduce themselves by dividing.	Reproduction of some of the lower forms of life is by d*******.	Dying Dividing Multiplying

5. Some lower forms of life (e.g. Hydra) reproduce by budding.	B**d*** is another way in which lower forms of life reproduce.	Branching Dividing Budding

6. These lower forms of life have no sex. Their reproduction is called **Asexual** reproduction.	Reproduction of forms of life which have no sex is called A**x*** reproduction.	Accidental Asexual Budding
7. **Asexual** reproduction does not require male and female sexes for it to take place.	If male and female sexes are not needed for reproduction it is called *se**** reproduction	Accidental Budding Fertilizing Asexual
8. The higher forms of life are in two sexes, male and female.	Two s****, male and female, are found in the higher forms of life.	Sexes Sorts Sizes
9. The female sex produces the egg cell.	E** c**** are produced by the female sex.	Ovules Egg cells Excuses
10. The female egg cell is called an **Ovum**.	An o*** is the name of a female egg cell.	Sperm Ovum Corpuscle

11. A lot of egg cells are called **Ova**.	Ova is the name for a lot of e** c****	Eggshells Eggcups Egg cells
12. The male sex produces a cell called a **Sperm**.	A *p**m cell is produced by the male sex.	Stuff Special Sperm
13. Before an egg cell will grow it must be **Fertilized** by a sperm cell.	Fertilization of an egg cell can only be done by a s**** cell.	Platelet Super Sperm
14. **Fertilization** means that the sperm cell actually burrows into the egg cell.	The sperm cell b****** into the egg cell to carry out fertilization.	Follows Burrows Borrows
15. Each egg cell is fertilized by only one sperm cell.	Only one ***** cell can fertilize an egg cell.	Pollen Corpuscle Sperm
16. Only one sperm cell can actually burrow into, and fertilize, each egg cell.	Burrowing into, and f*********** of, each egg cell is done by only one sperm cell.	
17. If an egg cell is fertilized it divides, and goes on dividing, until a new being is formed.	After fertilization, the egg cell d****** and goes on dividing.	Multiplies Disappears Divides
18. The new being, before birth, is called an **Embryo**.	The unborn being is known as an em****.	Elbow Embryo Baby
19. An **Embryo** is an unborn being, growing inside its mother, or inside an egg.	An unborn being is an **b***.	Egg cell Placenta Embryo
20. The fertilization of egg cells is done in several different ways.	Egg cells may be f********* in many ways.	Fertilized Farrowed Found

155

21. In reptiles, birds and mammals egg cells are fertilized **Inside** the female's body.	Egg cells are fertilized ****** the female's body, in birds, reptiles and mammals.	Outside Behind Below Inside
22. Fishes' eggs are fertilized by the male, after they have been laid by the female.	The male fish fertilizes eggs ***** they are laid.	While After Before
23. In reptiles, birds and mammals the male must place the sperm cells inside the female's body.	Sperm cells have to be placed inside the female's body by the ****.	Mate Male Mammal
24. In reptiles and birds, the embryo develops outside the body in an egg.	Reptiles and birds lay eggs and the embryo in the egg develops outside the ******'* body.	Fishes' Tortoise Female's
25. In mammals, the embryo develops inside the female's body.	The embryo develops inside the female's body, in **m****.	Mammals Males Mice
26. Mammal's babies are born alive.	Mammals give b**** to their young alive.	Lay Birth Born
27. Where male sperm cell and female egg cell are needed to produce young, this is called **sexual** reproduction.	Reproduction which need sperm and egg cell together is called S*****.	Sexual Asexual Bisexual Doubled

End of Programme . . . . Do Post-test

Programme S9B

1. Read the information in column A.
2. Complete the sentence in column B by choosing a word or number from Column C.
3. **Write out the whole sentence for your notes—do not write on the programme.**

4. Check answers from check list.
5. Do post-test (Do not write on the post-test paper).
6. Check answers to post-test.

Anatomy of Reproduction

A	B	C
Read this	**Complete this**	**Choose one of these to complete B**
1. The reproductive organs of all mammals are very similar.	Mammals have s***lar organs of reproduction.	Sexual Similar Several
2. Human beings are mammals.	Human beings belong to the group called m******.	Mums Monkeys Mammals
3. In women the reproductive organs are low down in the abdomen.	Reproductive organs are low down in the abdomen in **m*n.	Women Semen Pregnant

4.

Fallopian tube
Uterus
Vagina
Ovary

5. The ovaries produce the egg cells or ova.	The **a or egg cells are produced in the ovaries.	Oxo Ova Eggs
6. The tubes carry ova to the uterus.	Ova are carried to the u****s through tubes.	Eggs Ducts Uterus

7. If Ova are fertilized this happens in the tubes.	If fertilization of *** takes place it happens in the tubes.	Ovules Ovaries Ova
8. The tubes are called Fallopian Tubes.	The tubes which carry ova from *v*ries to uterus are the Fallopian tubes.	Uterine Ovulation Ovaries
9. The Fallopian tubes join the ovaries to the uterus.	The ovaries are joined to the uterus by the F***op**n tubes.	Fallopian Leucocyte Phallus
10. The tubes carrying ova from ovaries to uterus are the Fallopian tubes.	The **ll***an tubes carry ova from ovaries to uterus.	Parallel Fallopian Fertile
11. The uterus is often called the womb.	Another name for the womb is the ut***s.	Useless Uterus Genital
12. The womb is another name for the uterus.	The uterus is often called the **mb.	Tomb Womb Bomb
13. A passage leads from the uterus to an opening between the legs.	The uterus leads to a p****ge which opens between the legs.	Passage Plunge Penis
14. The passage from the uterus to the opening between the legs is called the vagina.	The v**in* is the passage from the uterus which opens between the legs.	Vulva Ova Vagina
15. The vagina is a passage leading to the uterus.	Leading to the uterus from an opening between the legs is a passage called the **g*n*.	Penis Vagina Virgin
16. The vagina opens into a cleft between the legs.	A cleft is between the girl's or woman's legs and the v***** opens into this cleft.	Vagina Vulva Vein

17. This cleft consists of thick folds of flesh called lips.	The vagina opens into thick fleshy lips forming a c**f*.	Cleft Curve Crutch
18. The cleft is called the vulva	The vulva is the proper name for the *le**.	Flesh Cleft Vagina
19. The opening out of which urine comes is also in the vulva.	The vulva also contains the opening from which u**ne comes.	Faeces Uterus Urine
20. Urine comes from another opening in the vulva.	Urine leaves another opening in the **lv*.	Vagina Vulva Fallopian
21. Hair covers the vulva in older girls and women.	In older girls and women the vulva is covered by h***.	No cue
22. Older girls and women also have breasts.	Breasts can be seen on older girls and w****.	No cue
23. The male reproductive organs are mainly outside the abdomen.	Outside the abdomen can be seen the m*** reproductive organs.	Minor Female Male

24.

Bladder

Sperm tube

Testis

Penis

25. Sperms are produced by the testicles.	The t**tic*** produce sperms.	Testicles Textiles Vulva
26. The testicles are also called the testes.	Another name for testicles is t*****.	Penis Tubes Testes
27. The testes are held in a skin bag which hangs between the legs.	Hanging between the legs and containing the testes is a skin ***.	No cue.
28. The testes are held in a skin bag.	A skin bag holds the t***es.	Tubes Testes Penis
29. The skin bag is called the scrotum.	The s*ro*** is the skin bag holding the testes.	Scrotum Scrofula Scapula
30. Sperms travel from the scrotum through a tube to the penis.	A tube along which sperms travel leads from the *cr**** to the penis.	Sternum Scrotum Testes
31. The penis is a fleshy tube which hangs down over the scrotum.	The fleshy tube hanging down over the scrotum is called the *en**.	Penis Testes Tendon
32. Both urine and sperms come out of the hole at the top of the penis.	Out of the hole in the top of the ***is come both urine and sperms.	Testes Penis Testicles
33. Urine and sperms cannot come out of the penis at the same time.	The hole in the penis will not pass urine and s***** at the same time.	Sternum Scapula Sperms
34. In older boys and men hair grows on the abdomen above the penis.	Hair grows on the abdomen above the p**** in older boys and men.	Veins Back Penis

35. Older boys and men do not have breasts.	Breasts do not grow on older boys and ***.	No cue

Programme S9C

1. Read the information in column A.
2. Complete the sentence in column B by choosing a word or number from Column C.
3. **Write out the whole sentence for your notes—do not write on the programme.**
4. Check answers from check list.
5. Do post-test (Do not write on the post-test paper).
6. Check answers to post-test.

Physiology of Reproduction

A	B	C
Read this	**Complete this**	**Choose one of these to complete B**
1. The testicles of a man produce sperm cells.	S***m cells are produced by the testicles of a man.	System Sperm Sexual
2. The ovaries of a woman produce ova.	Ova are produced by the ov***** of a woman.	Ovules Ovulation Ovaries
3. All mammals have either testicles or ovaries.	Testicles or ovaries are possessed by all m*mm***.	Mammals Mummies Monkeys
4. All male mammals have a penis.	A p**** is possessed by all male mammals.	Hairy Chest Penis Deep Voice
5. All female mammals have a vagina.	A v***** is possessed by all female mammals.	Vagina Virgin Daughter
6. A sperm must fertilize an ovum before the ovum will divide.	An ovum will divide only after being fertilized by a *p*r*.	Male Sperm Testicle

7. The ovum divides and goes on dividing.	Dividing of the o*** goes on after fertilization.	Gone Ovum Uterus
8. Eventually the dividing ovum will grow into a baby.	A baby will eventually develop from the dividing *v**.	Cells Ovum Venue
9. If a sperm is to fertilize the ovum it must be placed as near to the ovum as possible.	A sperm has to be placed closed to an ovum if f***il****ion is to take place.	Fertilization Fossilization Fumigation
10. To enable this the penis is placed inside the vagina.	The *en** has to be put inside the vagina.	Vas Deferens Glans Penis
11. So that sperm can be placed close to an ova the penis has to be put into the vagina.	The v****a needs to have the penis placed inside it if fertilization is to take place.	Venal Vagina Vestal
12. The penis is usually soft and hangs down over the scrotum.	The fleshy tube called the penis hangs down over the s***t*m.	Scrotum Scrofula Prepuce
13. The scrotum is a skin bag beneath the penis.	The penis hangs down over the s******.	Sacrom Scrotum Scapula
14. So that the penis can be placed inside the vagina it becomes stiff and rigid.	To enable the penis to be placed inside the **g**a it becomes stiff and rigid.	Angina Vagina Vein
15. So that the penis can be placed as far as possible into the vagina, the man and woman have to lie very close together.	The man and woman must lie very close together so that the **n** will be placed as far as possible into the vagina.	Puberty Sperm Penis

16. Other mammals have to get very close together, too.	Not only human beings need to get close together, but so do other *****ls.	Animals Mammals Horses
17. This getting close together is called sexual intercourse.	Sexual intercourse means the male places his penis inside the female's ******.	Test Tube Vas Deferens Vagina
18. Sometimes sexual intercourse is called mating.	Mating is another word for sexual **ter******.	Intercourse International Internment
19. Mating or intercourse is also called copulation.	Another word for m****g is copulation.	Marking Moving Mating
20. The getting close together is sometimes called copulation.	C**ul***** is another word for mating.	Calculation Copulation Consulation
21. Sperms pass from the tip of the penis into the vagina.	When the penis is in the vagina s***** come from the tip of it.	Saliva Sperms Corpuscles
22. From the vagina, sperms swim into the uterus.	Sperms leave the penis in the vagina and swim into the ut****.	Uterus Ovula Union
23. Sperms swim from the uterus into the Fallopian tubes.	From the uterus sperms swim into the Fall***** tubes.	Fallacious Freudism Fallopian
24. Sperms find their way into the Fallopian tubes from the uterus using their tails.	Using their tails, sperms swim into the Fallopian tubes from the *****s.	Hormones Humerus Uterus
25. Fertilization takes place in one of the Fallopian tubes.	It is in the Fallopian tubes that f***il****ion takes place.	Fallopian Fertilization Farination

26. Fertilization is a sperm burrowing into an ovum.	If a sperm burrows into an ovum this is called ***t*l*****on.	Fraternisation Pollination Fertilization

This is a long programme; break here and return to the programme later.

27. Usually only one ovum is fertilized by a sperm.	Only one sperm fertilizes only one ****.	Ovum Egg Ovule
28. Only one sperm can fertilize an ovum.	Each ovum is fertilized by only one *p***.	Cell Corpuscle Sperm
29. Sometimes two ova are fertilized by two sperms.	Occasionally two sperms may fertilize two ***.	Eggs Womb Ova
30. If two eggs are fertilized fraternal (unlike) twins will develop.	Fraternal tw*** develop if two eggs are fertilized.	Triplets Quads Twins
31. If a fertilized ovum splits into two separate halves, and these develop separately, identical (like) twins develop.	Identical twins develop if a fertilized o*** splits into two separate halves and each half develops separately.	Ovaries Ovum Ovulation
32. After fertilization the ovum passes into the uterus.	The ovum passes into the u****s after fertilization.	Uterus Usual Uvula
33. The ovum beds itself into the wall of the uterus.	The wall of the uterus is waiting for the ****.	No cue
34. The uterus will have prepared itself to receive the ovum.	The ovum beds itself to the prepared wall of the ******.	No cue

35. The uterus prepares a rich lining of blood and food materials.	A rich lining of blood and food material has been prepared by the ******.	No cue
36. If the ovum is not fertilized within 48 hours of leaving the ovary, it will die.	The ovum will die within ** hours of leaving the ovary if it is not fertilized.	24 36 48 72
37. If the ovum is not fertilized it remains in the uterus for a while then passes out of the uterus.	The ovum leaves the uterus after a while if it has not been f*********.	Fossilized Fixed Fertilized
38. The special lining of the womb also passes out through the vagina.	The uterus also sheds the special l***** through the vagina.	Leaving Ovum Lining
39. In women and older girls this happens about once every 28 days.	About every ** days egg and lining leave the uterus.	56 100 14 28
40. This is called menstruation or the monthly period.	The passing out of the ovum and lining is called m*n*********.	Menopause Menstruation Mentality
41. Menstruation is often called the monthly period.	Another name for menstruation is the monthly p***od.	Period Birth Intercourse

End of programme . . . . do post-test

Appendix F

Filmstrips

1. For children from about seven to eleven.

Where Do Babies Come From? Made for Schools Broadcasting Council of BBC.

Programme consists of two parts:–

1. Coloured filmstrip 35mm. F256, including teachers' notes.
2. Radio commentary broadcast in *Nature Series* for schools to tape. Pupils' pamphlet for *Nature Series*. Tapes obtainable from BBC Publications. Tape and Notes T236.

Growing Up. Made for Schools Broadcasting Council of BBC. Programme consists of two parts.

1. Coloured filmstrip 35mm. F257, including teachers' notes.
2. Radio commentary broadcast in *Nature Series* for schools to tape. Tapes and Notes obtainable from BBC Publications. T237.

Let's Talk About Ourselves, No. 1, Camera Talks Ltd., 23 Denmark Place, WC2.

Consists of two parts.

1. Coloured filmstrip 35mm.
2. Tape.

Let's Talk About Ourselves, No. 2.
As above.

How Life is Handed On. C.Ga.340. Cyril Bibby. Common Ground, Ltd., 44 Fulham Road, SW3.
Black-and-white 35mm. filmstrip with teachers' notes.

Other Material.
Works cards. *How Life Begins.* Published by James Galt.
Model of Visible Woman. Renival (U.S.).
Model of Visible Man. Renival (U.S.).

2. For children of about eleven to thirteen.
Human Reproduction. Schools Broadcasting Council. BBC Programme consists of two parts.
1. Filmstrip. 35mm. F2.88 with notes.
2. Radio commentary broadcast in 'Life Cycle' for schools to tape.

Inside the Body. Programme consists of two parts. Extra copy of notes H289.
1. Filmstrip 35mm. F289. With notes.
2. Radio commentary broadcast in Life Cycle for schools to tape.
Man and Woman. Part 1. 8mm. film loop. 4 mins. Camera Talks.
Man and Woman. Part 2. 8mm. film loop. 4 mins. Camera Talks.

BBC materials available from:
BBC Publications, 35 Marylebone High Street, London, W1.

Appendix G

Films

There are few 16mm films made for young children. The most child-centred are films of television programmes.

1. Beginnings ⎱ Three 16mm. films of the series which appears
2. Birth ⎰ annually in the BBC education programme
3. Full Circle ⎰ 'Merry-Go-Round' for about eight- to ten-year-olds.

Obtainable from BBC Publications, 35 Marylebone High Street, London, W1.

Eight programmes in the series 'Living and Growing' made by Grampian Television for ten to thirteen-year-olds may be made available as 16mm. films for purchase.

Enquiries to Grampian Television Ltd., Queen's Cross, Aberdeen, AB9 2XS.

Material for Older Pupils in Secondary Schools.

Starting points for discussion in the field of personal relationships.

1. Film Loops. 8mm. Numerous titles. Camera Talks, Ltd.
2. BBC Radio Programmes for taping in schools. (Teachers are strongly advised to listen to the programme first before using with pupils.)

Learning About Life for fourteen- to sixteen-year-olds. Long-playing record available from BBC Radio Enterprises, London, SE19. Pupils' pamphlets essential. P107, N107.

Inquiry. Fourteen- to sixteen-year-olds.
3. BBC Television for Schools. *Scene* provides talking points for fifteen- to sixteen-year-olds on subjects directly related to contemporary life.

Schools Council Projects Teaching Material.
Humanities Curriculum Project (Heinemann Educational):
'The Family'
'Relationships between the Sexes'

Moral Education Curriculum Project (Longman):
General Guide: 'Moral Education in the Secondary School'
Set 1: 'In Other People's Shoes'
Set 2: 'Proving the Rule'
Set 3: 'What Would You Have Done?'

170

Index

Other titles in the Evans Modern Teaching series

Resources in Schools by R. P. A. Edwards describes the nature and use of the school resource centre: how it can be designed, administered and staffed, its library, audio-visual and retrieval functions, and its central role in the life and work of the school. Numerous illustrations show apparatus and existing resource centres in operation.

School in the Town by Barbara Blit looks at environmental studies as a developing part of the primary and middle school curriculum. It is written particularly for teachers of children in the 8 to 13 age range, and offers a practical programme full of useful ideas for the study of their environment by children in urban and suburban areas.

Parent-teacher Partnership by Graham Bond poses fundamental questions regarding the desirability of parent-teacher co-operation. The author, who is a recognised authority in the field, discusses beliefs and attitudes, considers the many problems met by teachers and parents, and offers ideas and solutions which vary according to the different backgrounds of the people concerned.

History with Juniors by Michael Pollard outlines a modern approach towards teaching history to junior and middle school children. Various projects are discussed, always in practical terms, including the use of archive material, local history sources and field work, and the author describes the relationship between such projects and other curriculum areas.

Sums for Today by Gordon Pemberton presents a cogent argument in favour of the new methods of teaching elementary mathematics, using concrete, structured materials. The author establishes that traditional methods, stemming from practices of Victorian ledger-clerks, are irrelevant to today's situation, and give the learner little understanding of the concepts of calculation. He also establishes, using many illustrated examples, that the new methods are mathematically based, essentially practical and easy to understand.

have
(5) Sex Education